"FIRST DO NO HARM..."

"FIRST DO NO HARM..."

A Dying Woman's Battle Against the
Physicians and Drug Companies Who
Misled Her About the Hazards of THE PILL

Natalee S. Greenfield

SUN RIVER PRESS
TWO CONTINENTS PUBLISHING GROUP, LTD.

Library of Congress Cataloging in Publication Data

Greenfield, Natalee S
    "First do no harm . . . ."

    1.   Products liability—Drugs—United States.
2.   Malpractice—United States.   3.   Breast—Cancer.
I.   Title.
KF1297.D7G7   346'.73'038   76-20629
ISBN 0-8467-0198-7

Copyright © 1976 by Natalee S. Greenfield

Acknowledgements

    The author is grateful for permission to quote from *The Washington Post* from
articles by Morton Mintz, Victor Cohn and Nicholas Von Hoffman; *United Press
International; Newsweek; The New York Times* from articles by Boyce
Rensberger, Theodore Shabad and others; and Bell-McClure Syndicate from
columns by Drew Pearson and Jack Anderson.

    Deep appreciation and gratitude is expressed to Dr. Herbert Ratner, editor of
Child and Family Quarterly. Dr. Ratner is a brilliant physician, dedicated public
servant, and great humanitarian who dares to demand that his fellow physicians
follow the motto of their esteemed profession, "First Do No Harm . . ."

Production by Planned Production
Text design by Joyce C. Weston
Printed in USA
Two Continents Publishing Group, Ltd.
30 East 42 Street
New York NY 10017
and Sun River Press

346.038
G8/2

The story set forth in this narrative is true. Names have been changed because of
legal restrictions.

Dedicated to my Daughter
who was the "Kathryn" of this book

Foreword

It must be emphasized in this area of consumer protection, that the woman has a right to protection from manipulation and victimization. No right is more firmly established than the right of the patient to informed consent to a prescription directed at his body, whether surgical or medicinal. Knowledge sufficient for enlightened consent is a moral, medical and legal right to which malpractice suits testify. The classic statement of this right is found in Plato's Laws . . . where Plato distinguishes between the physician who took care of slaves, and the one who took care of freemen. Whereas the slave-doctor prescribed "as if he had exact knowledge" and gave orders "like a tyrant" the doctors of freemen went "into the nature of the disorder," entered "into discourse with the patient and his friends" and would not "prescribe for him until he has first convinced him." The reader can determine for himself whether the American woman, as patient, is treated as slave or free person. It is our belief that the decline of responsibility to the individual patient in the area of family planning by groups and individuals working in this field is resulting in a national scandal.

Herbert Ratner, M.D.
Editor, Child & Family Quarterly
The Medical Hazards of the Birth Control Pill
Child and Family Reprint Booklet
Oak Park, Illinois 1969

"FIRST DO
NO HARM..."

Part One

"With the widespread use of the oral contraceptives—The Pill iatrogenic [physician-caused] disease has hit epidemic proportions. Up until now physicians, for the most part, have only been producing iatrogenic disease as a by-product of treating the already sick person. For the first time in medicine's history, however, the drug industry has placed at our disposal a powerful, disease-producing chemical for use in the healthy rather than the sick.

". . . Let there be no doubt about the medical dangers of The Pill. I think it sufficient to recognize that we never had congressional hearings on the safety of other methods of contraception control. . . ."

Herbert Ratner, M.D.
Editor, Child & Family Quarterly
The Medical Hazards of the Birth Control Pill
Child and Family Reprint Booklet
Oak Park, Illinois 1969

Chapter One

November 17, 1968.

Dillard Hospital resembled a well maintained old New York City hotel with a dining room that was known for its excellent cuisine.

After Kathryn completed filling out necessary forms at the reception desk, a young man took her overnight case and escorted her and her mother to a room on the ninth floor.

Kathryn unpacked her small bag and placed a picture of Julie, her toy-sized poodle, on the desk facing the bed. She tried to appear calm, sensing her mother's apprehension.

"Come on, Mommy," she said, as she brushed her forehead against Noreen's cheek, "they're only going to remove a little lump from your bump," she teased. "Noreen and her Bump" was the way Kathryn's mother had signed letters to her parents during her pregnancy.

Kathryn's father, Roy, arrived from the University with a big "Hi!" and kept the conversation light and relaxing. Roy had been a national A.A.U. champion in several sports during his college days, and his daughter had acquired some of his athletic prowess. She could bat a baseball over a rooftop, throw a hard ball a good distance and played a wicked game of tennis, pingpong and badminton.

There were no visiting hour regulations at Dillard Hospital, but there came a point when the hall lights were dimmed. Noreen kissed Kathryn goodnight and promised not to see her until after she was returned to her room from surgery the following day. Kathryn said it would be better for both of them.

The next day, some eight hours after surgery, Dr. Wilkinson finally made his appearance. His face was grim. "Mrs. Stuart," he said to Noreen, "in my thirty years of surgery, I have never seen such a strange tumor, nor have I ever had a breast cancer patient as young as Kathryn. I didn't do a radical mastectomy, even though the frozen section findings were positive. If your daughter was older, I would have. I want additional pathologists at Memorial Hospital to review the frozen section; we should have their findings tomorrow. However, there's no doubt in my mind that a radical mastectomy is indicated. Of course, we will wait to see what the final reports show."

Noreen was very much shaken by his comments. Her worst fears had been realized. She took several moments to gather her thoughts. "Dr. Wilkinson," she said slowly, "I really don't know what to say. Kathryn and her husband must make the final decision. I'll discuss it with my husband. . . ."

He cut her off. "It's important that we don't delay surgery any longer than we have to." There was undisguised urgency in his voice.

Kathryn was returned to her room and slept most of the day. Occasionally she opened her eyes and smiled at her mother. A feeling of impending doom overwhelmed Noreen. This was her child, in danger of her life.

Home from the hospital, Noreen telephoned a few of her closest friends who were physicians. They all said the same thing: it was unheard of for a woman to have breast cancer at Kathryn's age. They urged Noreen to check the diagnosis, and see that the pathologists hadn't confused the results of Kathryn's biopsy with those of someone else's.

Dr. Wilkinson arranged for a meeting with Kathryn's parents at the hospital the next day. Kathryn's husband, Conrad, had to attend a seminar at a medical school; he said he couldn't be there. Dr. Wilkinson told the Stuarts that the pathologists' final reports showed that Kathryn's tumor was malignant. Their daughter should have her breast removed at once.

No, absolutely, there had been no mix-up in the laboratory findings. He had examined the tissues himself to make certain there was no error. He asked the Stuarts to join him when he explained the need for surgery to Kathryn. She was waiting for her parents in her hospital room.

The doctor greeted Kathryn warmly. He sat down on the bed next to her and placed his large, strong hand over hers. He told her exactly what he had said to her parents. "There's no other way, Kathryn," he concluded.

Kathryn, trying to stay calm, listened intently. But there was terror in her eyes when she turned to her parents. She seemed to be waiting for someone to tell her that it was a bad joke—perhaps she was having a nightmare? It *couldn't* be happening to *her*! No one in her family ever had cancer. . . .

Her parents seemed to be pinned against the wall, speechless.

Finally Kathryn said, "And I was worried about having a little scar on my breast. . . . Now I'll be disfigured. . . ."

The doctor reassured her. She'd be as good as new after the radical. Kathryn wanted very much to believe him. She watched him as he got up and started to leave.

She glanced toward the three of them and in a pleading, trembling voice said, "I don't want to die. . . ." A tear trickled from the corner of her almond-shaped eye. "I don't want to lose my breast either," she said, barely above a whisper, as her hand automatically went to her left breast. "But . . .," she took a deep breath, "but above all. . . , I don't want to die. . . !"

The next day, Wednesday, the anesthesiologist put Kathryn to sleep for the second time in three days, and the surgery began.

Hours later, Dr. Wilkinson joined Kathryn's parents in the waiting room.

"Kathryn will be down from the operating room in a few hours," he told them. "The operation was uneventful. Everything looks clean. I believe I took out the entire malignancy the other day when I removed the tumor, but I can't say definitely until the tissues that we took out today are analyzed. It will take about two weeks for us to have a final answer."

After Dr. Wilkinson left them, he went into his office and wrote the following for Kathryn's file:

Admission Date: 11/17/68

Huffman, Kathryn

Dillard Hospital #11745

Kathryn Stuart Huffman was originally seen at the office of Dr. Julius Wilkinson on November 2, 1968. She was 22 years of age at that time and she stated that in the preceding April, she had taken a birth control pill, Cyclemide, for a period of three months time, but she was quite unhappy with its side effects. In August, she was subjected to examination again and she stated that her breasts were considered normal at that time by the examining gynecologist and she was put on Mordrine as a birth control measure. Soon after this time, a nodule appeared in the left breast.

When we examined her, she had a 2 cm. nodule in the central zone of the axillary segment of the left breast. It did not transilluminate clearly, but there was no axillary adenopathy, and the right breast was normal. We felt that she had a fibroadenoma of the breast and suggested that she be admitted to the hospital to have this excised. She was admitted to Dillard Hospital and on November 18, under general anesthesia, a local excision examination was done. We were quite surprised that the diagnosis was returned as medullary cancer with lymphoid infiltration.

We did not do the radical mastectomy that day and asked for careful review of permanently prepared frozen sections, and the following day the diagnosis was sustained in that manner.

The matter was discussed with Kathryn and her family and we told her that this particular lesion had an excellent prognosis as far as serious tumors of the breast were concerned as there were lymphocytes surrounding the tumor, yet she must have a radical mastectomy.

She assented to that operation which was done on November 20, 1968. The pathological report at that time did not show any metastasis to the regional lymph nodes and there was no residual after the previous excision.

All of which meant that Dr. Wilkinson, much to his surprise, had found Kathryn's breast tumor to be cancerous, but that he had no reason to think it had spread or that he hadn't removed the tumor entirely. To be absolutely safe, he had removed the affected breast.

Kathryn was not returned to her room until some twelve hours later. She hadn't yet opened her eyes, but she was not sleeping peacefully. On the bedpost bottles of glucose and plasma were hung, providing nourishment, feeding into her right arm. Her left hand was wrapped tightly in an elastic bandage that led up to her shoulder and across her chest.

Arrangements had been made for private nurses around the clock. Kathryn was helpless. She could not use either hand.

She continually tossed her head from side to side, crying out, "Help me! Help me!" Later she recalled a nightmare that kept repeating itself:

There was a warrior standing in a battlefield with the bodies of beautiful women lying around him on the blood-soaked ground.

The warrior looked like Dr. Wilkinson—and she, Kathryn, was his last victim. In one hand there was a sword raised high, blood dripping from it; in the other, a silver tray held triumphantly over his head, garnished with the breasts he had sliced from the other bodies. While blood gushed from holes in the women's chests, he cheered, "I am a Brave Victorious Warrior!"

One of Kathryn's first visitors was a patient from across the hall. To her great surprise, it was a man: a priest named Father Jude. Kathryn's room was on a floor reserved for breast surgery cases, and she expected to find only women there. Father Jude was recovering from his second radical mastectomy.

"Well, at least you can't blame your breast cancer on the birth control pill," Kathryn said jokingly.

Father Jude sighed. "That's not quite so," he said. "I have a prostate condition, and I was given the female hormone, estrogen, for it. It's the same hormone that's in the birth control pill, and I'm told that's what brought on my breast cancer."

Kathryn paled. "You were told that the estrogen hormone caused your breast cancer? I suspect that the estrogen in the birth control pill triggered *my* breast cancer. As soon as I get home I'm going to ask a lot of people a lot of questions!"

On Thanksgiving Day, Kathryn was discharged from the hospital. Before leaving she stopped by Father Jude's room and promised to keep in touch with him.

Chapter Two

November 30, 1968.

Kathryn went to the local drugstore and asked the druggist, Mr. Logan, if he had any literature concerning the birth control pill. He gave her a leaflet printed by a pharmaceutical company. She read it before she left the pharmacy. In it she found some information pertinent to her condition:

SIDE EFFECTS OBSERVED IN PATIENTS RECEIVING ORAL CONTRACEPTIVES

The following *adverse reactions* have been observed with varying incidence in patients receiving oral contraceptives:

Nausea	Spotting
Vomiting	Change in menstrual flow
Gastrointestinal symptoms	Breast changes
Breakthrough bleeding	Amenorrhea
Edema	Rash
Migraine	Mental depression

CONTRAINDICATIONS

1. Patients with thrombophlebitis or with a history of thrombophlebitis or pulmonary embolism [blood clots].

2. Liver dysfunction or disease.
3. Patients with known or suspected carcinoma of breasts or genital organs.

"And they told me The Pill was as safe as aspirin!" Kathryn said to the pharmacist. "Aspirin doesn't cause breast cancer. How does one know that she's prone to breast cancer? Why wasn't I given this literature to read *before* I took The Pill?"

"The American Medical Association and the drug firms don't want this information shared with the patient," Mr. Logan explained.

From the Record
The *Evening Record*, January 22, 1970.*

A doctor-turned-lawyer told Congress today that birth control pills were deviously promoted to lessen the bad news impact of their harmful effects on both physicians and their patients.

The accusation was made by J. Harold Williams, Berkeley, California, who gave up the practice of medicine in 1960 to represent patients in malpractice suits against doctors.

The Senate antimonopoly subcommittee called Williams to testify during a second week of hearings on oral contraceptives. About nine million American women take The Pill.

"Sometimes the physician is unsuspectingly caught in the middle betweeen his conscientious desire to serve his patients and intensive promotional pressure by drug manufacturers.

"The sad saga of The Pill is one of the most pheno-

*United Press International

menal examples of such an entrapment," Williams said.

"Doctors," Williams said, "rely on pharmaceutical companies for much, if not all, information about drugs. He [the doctor] assumes that the drug companies are honest and that the Food and Drug Administration has been a vigilant watchdog to protect him and his patients.

"Some prominent doctors have promoted The Pill, often with denials of its dangers," Dr. Williams said, "and often with irrelevant analogies and misstatements of fact. . . .

December 2, 1968.

Kathryn had asked her mother to drive her to the medical library at the College of Physicians and Surgeons, Columbia University's medical school. There she found accounts of the many ways in which The Pill could affect a person's health. One could spend years just studying about different ways The Pill attacks some vital organs and various diseases it can trigger. Kathryn limited her reading to breast cancer. The following points were made repeatedly in cancer journals:

● It has been known since 1898 that hormones affect breast cancer.

● The hormone estrogen, which is used in the birth control pill, may stimulate the growth of breast cancer even if administered in small doses.

● All animals given estrogen over a period of time in laboratory tests developed breast cancer.

● Breast cancer research with these animals is applicable to humans.

● The argument that estrogen has not increased the incidence of breast cancer in older women at the time of menopause does not apply to young women who are still menstruating and producing their own estrogen.

December 12, 1968.
Kathryn saw a story in *The New York Times*:*

> MOSCOW, Dec. 11—Soviet public health officials have decided to begin mass manufacture of intrauterine devices in preference to contraceptive pills.
>
> Dr. Boris Petrovsky, Minister of Public Health, disclosed the Government's decision in a letter to the weekly newspaper, *Literaturnaya Gazeta* published today.
>
> The choice of the most effective modern contraceptive has been a major problem for Soviet authorities. . . .
>
> Discussing contraceptive pills, Dr. Petrovsky said, "As far as hormonal preparations are concerned, they are unlikely to be used widely because they can produce undesirable side effects and sometimes serious complications."

December 13, 1968.
Kathryn wanted to share her concern about The Pill with someone in a position to do something about it. She called the American Cancer Society. The Vice President of the Society happened to answer the phone. The following conversation took place:

"Doctor, I'd like to make an appointment to speak with you about the possible connection between birth control pills and breast cancer."

"I can tell you right now that there is absolutely no evidence to show that any connection exists."

"I'm not calling to *ask* about The Pill. I'm calling to report my own experience with it. Soon after I started to take these pills I got sick. Three months later I found a growth in my breast that was later found to be cancerous."

"That's too bad!"

*Theodore Shabad, *The New York Times*, Dec. 12, 1968.

"Doctor, isn't there something that can be done to warn people about the risks they may run by taking The Pill? Their physicians usually assure them that there is no risk. But that's not true! Don't you want cases like mine reported? Doesn't that kind of information help the research effort in this area?"

"If I were you, Mrs. Huffman, I wouldn't worry about warning or helping other people. You are obviously 'cancer-prone.' Just worry about yourself. Spend your time watching out for a possible reoccurrence."

"Tell me Doctor, do you have any daughters?"

"I have two."

"What, if anything, have you told them about The Pill?"

There was a pause.

"I advised them not to take it."

"Why?"

"I'm afraid that birth control pills may not be good for their health."

Chapter Three

December 14, 1968, 3:00 P.M.

Kathryn, accompanied by her mother, went for her first post-operative visit to Dr. Wilkinson at his office. After waiting two hours, she was admitted to his examining room.

Dr. Wilkinson came in, greeted his patient warmly, and changed the dressing on her wound. It was a 12-inch incision extending from Kathryn's left shoulder blade to her midriff. There was another large open hole under her left armpit.

After Dr. Wilkinson removed the stitches, he wiped the dried blood from the wound and applied a fresh dressing. He then rewrapped Kathryn's arm and chest with an elastic bandage, leaving her right breast exposed.

As the doctor began to palpate her right breast, Kathryn asked in a half-joking, half-serious manner, "Looking for more business, Dr. Wilkinson?"

"Put on your blouse and come into my office. I want to talk to you," he said. He brushed a lock of Kathryn's hair from near her eye and left the room.

As the two women re-entered Wilkinson's office, Kathryn said, "Oh, yes, before I forget, I need some more percodan. I took the last one you gave me today."

"You shouldn't be taking percodan any more," he replied. "Dr. Wilkinson, I need it. I really do. I have a lot of pain. I can't even straighten up because of the pain. It's all through the left side of my body. It starts in my left shoulder and goes all the way down my side and across my chest."

"Very well, I'll give you a prescription for one week's supply. But that's it! I don't want you to become addicted to percodan." He wrote out a new prescription and handed it to her.

"I just received the laboratory report with the analysis of tissues removed from your breast and lymph nodes," he went on. "The results are negative. That means the malignancy was actually removed when I took out the tumor during the first surgery. It had not spread through your breast, or under your arm. There's no need for any further treatment, such as cobalt therapy."

"Are you saying that the whole cancer was removed and contained in the small nodule you took out on the 18th? That I didn't have to have my breast removed two days later?" Kathryn exclaimed.

Dr. Wilkinson frowned. "The malignancy was removed on the 18th, yes," he said. "But it was imperative to have the radical mastectomy. Otherwise, you never would have had peace of mind, not knowing whether we'd actually gotten the cancer."

"But I *don't* have peace of mind! My breast is gone!" Tears filled Kathryn's eyes. "And if the cancer has been removed, why do I feel so ill? You seem to think I shouldn't be having all this pain. Why hasn't the wound healed more?"

Dr. Wilkinson was obviously at a loss for an answer.

Kathryn burst out, "My husband said the wound should have been almost healed by now. He wanted to have intercourse with me and it hurt me so much when he touched my body, I had to make him stop! He was angry! He said there was no medical reason for me not to have intercourse with him."

"I don't understand either why you're having so much pain and difficulty," Dr. Wilkinson admitted.

"Please, Dr. Wilkinson, would you meet with my husband and tell him that I'm not ready for sexual relations with him yet? He thinks I'm rejecting him on purpose."

"I really couldn't do that, because I see no reason why you shouldn't have intercourse with him now. It's important for you to do everything you did before the surgery. You're not fragile or an invalid! Why, in no time you'll be back on the tennis court."

"You just don't understand how miserable I feel," Kathryn said.

Dr. Wilkinson stood up, "Kathryn, I would like to see you three times a week until your incision is healed. See my nurse and make your next appointment."

Conrad, Kathryn's husband, had been unreasonable and estranged from her since her breast had been removed. Maybe he didn't want a wife with one breast. Breasts were important to him.

December 19, 1968.

Kathryn had written a letter to the United States Food and Drug Administration:

> In the *McCall's* November 1968 article about the birth control pill, it said the FDA had announced that birth control packages will have to be labeled with a warning that the pills may be hazardous to one's health.
>
> Would you please advise me what steps, if any, have been taken by the FDA to activate this plan?
>
> Sincerely yours,
> Kathryn Stuart Huffman

March 6, 1969, 2:00 A.M. Home of Kathryn's parents.

Kathryn's grandmother screamed. Her parents ran from their bedroom. Kathryn's grandmother was in the hall by the open bathroom door. Kathryn was huddled on the bathroom floor, white and shivering, retching violently into the toilet, unable to stop. Her incision was ripped open, blood soaked her pajama top. As her father kneeled down to her, she fainted in his arms.

At 2:30 A.M. Roy finally reached Dr. Wilkinson by phone. He would see Kathryn at 3:00 that afternoon.

March 7, 1969, 3:00 P.M.

Dr. Wilkinson gave Kathryn a thorough examination and changed her dressing. "Everything appears to be all right. You no doubt have a virus."

Kathryn gasped, "Dr. Wilkinson, I can't go on this way! It's March 7th now. I was operated on nearly four months ago! My incision hasn't healed. I'm in constant pain all through my left side—especially in my left shoulder! I have been seeing you three times a week for the past four months. You keep working on this incision and it doesn't do any good!"

"The only thing I can think of," the doctor said, "was that I did a 'thin fold' stitch so that there wouldn't be a thick scar. If you can visualize a tailor sewing a seam and taking just enough material so the seam won't be unattractive, that's what I did with your incision."

"It's inconceivable to me how you could be so concerned about the aesthetic appearance of the scar when the surgery left my chest and armpit completely deformed," she cried.

"I did what I thought was in your best interest," Dr. Wilkinson replied. "Perhaps if I did a thicker fold it would hold together. Would you be willing for me to operate again?"

"I'd be willing for anything that will make me heal!"

"On second thought, let's try something else before we rush into more surgery. I'd like you to apply a solution of salt water to your wound every hour."

When she reached home, Kathryn phoned Dr. Aaron. "You referred me to Dr. Wilkinson. Now I'm asking you to refer me to someone else. I want my wound to heal. I can't stand its ripping apart, and having this constant pain."

"Very well, Kathryn. There's a man at University Hospital

who's from India. His name is Daniel Ashoka. Maybe with his technique he can help you. I'll phone him and discuss your case with him."

March 17, 1969. Home of Kathryn's parents.

Conrad issued an ultimatum to Kathryn: either she have intercourse with him within ten days or he'd have their marriage annulled.

His wife's anger rose. "A happy St. Patrick's Day to you, too!"

Chapter Four

March 19, 1969.

In her local paper, Kathryn read this in Drew Pearson's and Jack Anderson's syndicated column,*

Washington—Come May, the birth control pill will have been on the market for nine years. Yet the Food and Drug Administration is unable to say how many adverse reactions The Pill has caused during this period or how many deaths have been associated with its use.

The matter is so serious that two Congressional committees have been quietly investigating reports that at least ten per cent of all adverse reaction reports are fatalities and that one-third of the recent reports on one specific pill involve death. But no one can say with any certainty how high the death rate really is.

This column has learned that since October 1968 there are approximately 9,000 adverse reports covering the years 1965 and 1966 which have yet to be included in the overall total. These reports are still piled high in room 602-C at the Food and Drug Administration.

*Drew Pearson and Jack Anderson, Bell-McClure Syndicate.

Meanwhile, an estimated 7,000,000 American women are using The Pill. It works; but apparently in more ways than one.

So serious are the side effects reported by the British in April of last year that the Food and Drug Administration ordered American manufacturers to relabel, warning that English studies estimate "there is a 7-to-10-fold increase in mortality and morbidity due to thromboembolic (clotting in the blood vessels) diseases in women taking oral contraceptives. . . . Statistical evaluation indicated that the difference observed between users and non-users was highly significant."

This column has now learned, from a medical authority in a position to know, that independent American studies to be published this spring "fully confirm" the British studies.

It seems incredible, therefore, that if The Pill is not safe we should have to wait till the British tell us so.

So far The Pill has led a charmed life. The first Pill, called "Enovid," was passed by FDA on the basis that 132 women have received it continuously for a year or more. . . .

. . . FDA has now acknowledged to interested Congressmen that between January, 1966 and December 1, 1968, it had found reports of 1,023 "serious and fatal" cases of which 115 involved death and 908 were serious. Blood clots accounted for 84 of the deaths and 459 of the "serious" reactions, among which were listed cancer and hepatitis.

By no means were these a total of all adverse reactions reported, but only those FDA considered "serious and fatal," such as strokes. . . .

. . . FDA had no way of obtaining full reports of adverse reactions. True, the drug companies are required to report, but not the attending physician. And there is always the question as to the ultimate cause of death in the individual case."

March 27, 1969. Home of Kathryn's parents.

A letter for Kathryn. It was from a lawyer in New York City, and it said that he represented Conrad Huffman, who was initiating a divorce action against her. The lawyer offered her a free trip to Mexico, all expenses to be paid by Conrad, in exchange for a "quickie divorce."

Kathryn got in touch with a family friend who was a lawyer. "This is what I want you to do," Sam Groden said. "First, withdraw the money from your joint savings account. You'll need that as a partial payment toward a divorce lawyer's retainer fee. I'm not a divorce lawyer, but I'll handle your case in New Jersey until you find a lawyer in New York.

"Second," he went on, "I want your parents to cancel the lease they signed for your apartment immediately."

Eventually, and with reluctance, Kathryn complied with Sam's suggestions, only to learn that Conrad had already been at the bank and had tried to close both accounts. He wasn't successful since he did not have the passbooks.

March 31, 1969.

Kathryn officially changed her address from Englewood Cliffs to her parents' Short Hills home. She also phoned New Jersey Blue Cross-Blue Shield.

"I would like to transfer my hospital insurance to my name from my husband's name. We have a Family Plan Policy," she explained.

"Have your husband write a letter to that effect," the voice replied.

"But I have no contact with my husband. We're separated."

"Then we'll send you an application and you can apply as a single person," the voice continued.

"Do I need a physical examination? I just had a radical mastectomy."

"Oh, then you won't be acceptable for hospital or surgical insurance under our plan. I suggest you get your husband to drop us a note requesting the transfer. Then you will be completely covered, including your present medical problems, as a single policy holder."

May 31, 1969.

Sam Groden, Kathryn's lawyer, sent her copies of two letters he had received from Conrad's lawyer:

April 22, 1969
RE: *Conrad and Kathryn Huffman*
Dear Mr. Groden:

I would appreciate your letting me know what progress is being made toward arranging for a conference to discuss this matter.

While I have taken up the matter of arranging for separate Blue Cross and Blue Shield policies, I have not pressed this with my client, pending the proposed meeting.

Very truly yours,
Richard Cawley

May 29, 1969
RE: *Conrad and Kathryn Huffman*
Dear Mr. Groden:

I would appreciate your letting me know what progress is being made towards arranging for a conference to discuss this matter.

As I told you, the time is rapidly coming for payment of the medical and hospital insurance premiums. While I have taken up the matter of arranging for separate Blue Cross and Blue Shield policies, I have not pressed the matter with my client. We are all aware that your client is not eligible for coverage as a single person, as she will be unable to pass her physical examination. My client needs no coverage since he is a physician. Therefore, I will have to make a decision as to how to advise my client in view of the fact that your client is unwilling to get a Mexican divorce and claims she is not well enough to have sexual relations with her husband.

Very truly yours,
Richard Cawley

June 9, 1969. Sam Groden's office, Short Hills, N.J.

Sam asked Kathryn to come to his office to discuss the divorce action. "The time has come," Sam said, "when you will have to retain a New York lawyer. But let Conrad initiate the divorce action against you and then counter-sue on grounds of cruelty and abandonment."

He handed Kathryn some papers. "I ran off these copies of letters I received from his lawyer. They're for your file, along with my answers."

After Kathryn looked over the letters, Sam repeated, "The time has come for you to get a New York lawyer. Sylvia and I are leaving for Europe next week, and we won't be back until September. I was at the Harvard Club last night and I spoke to a few friends who gave me the names of some New York divorce lawyers for you. I ought to warn you—most of them charge a minimum of $3,500 as a retainer fee."

Kathryn winced. "That *is* steep! I've got so many medical and educational expenses. I have some friends who have lawyer cousins in New York. Maybe they can help us find a good lawyer who won't charge that much. And please, Sam, do send me your bill."

"All I want from you is for you to get entirely well, Kathryn," Sam said. "That will be my payment in full."

"Someday, someway, I'll repay you," Kathryn promised.

"Sam, before I leave, there's something else. Could you recommend a lawyer who specializes in malpractice suits?"

"Well, yes, as a matter of fact I can. One of my former Harvard classmates has a great reputation in that field. His name is Paul Slater, and he has an office in the Pan Am Building in New York."

"Maybe I'll call him one of these days," Kathryn said as she made a note of his name on a piece of paper. "May I say you recommended him?"

"By all means," Sam replied.

"Have a good summer," he said, seeing her out. "I'll contact you when we get back."

Chapter Five

June 12, 1969.

Kathryn received a letter and some printed material from the U.S. Department of Health, Education and Welfare:

> Congressman Fountain has referred to us his response to your letter of April 17, 1969, regarding your request for literature dealing with the safety of oral contraceptives.
>
> We are enclosing a copy of the August 1, 1966 FDA Report on the Oral Contraceptives. This report was prepared by the Advisory Committee on Obstetrics and Gynecology to the Food and Drug Administration in our continuing effort to evaluate the safety and effectiveness of these products.
>
> We believe the bibliography will supply information of interest to you.
>
> Additional information on the subject should be available from your medical library.
>
> > Sincerely yours,
> > Edwin M. Ortiz, M.D., Director
> > Division of Metabolic and
> >   Endocrine Drug Surveillance
> > Office of Market Drugs
> > Bureau of Medicine

Enclosed was this material, which the letter indicated was "to be carried on the 'package insert' for the information of the prescribing physician and the medical profession."

FDA FACT SHEET
ORAL CONTRACEPTIVES

"The oral contraceptives present society with problems unique in the history of human therapeutics," the Food and Drug Administration's Advisory Committee on Obstetrics and Gynecology noted in a report issued August, 1966. "Never will so many people have taken such potent drugs voluntarily over such a protracted period for an objective other than for the control of disease."

Perhaps because they are unique, there has been widespread public interest in the oral contraceptives. Many inquiries about the "birth-control" pills are received by the FDA. The FDA does not publish literature describing individual products, but this fact sheet provides general information about the entire class of drugs known as oral contraceptives.

All of the oral contraceptives are considered "new drugs" under the provisions of the Federal Food, Drug and Cosmetic Act. This means they must be proved both *safe* and *effective* when used as directed before permission for commercial distribution is granted by the FDA.

At this time, two types of oral contraceptives for females—combined and sequential—have been approved by the FDA. Both types of drugs contain chemical replicas of the natural hormones estrogen and progesterone; the combined type gives both hormones throughout the regimen of use and the sequential type gives only one hormone at the beginning of the regimen followed by a dosage of both hormones.

Oral contraceptives are available in various dosage strengths and under a number of different trade names.

The oral contraceptives have been cleared for marketing as prescription drugs, because medical supervision by a physician is a significant factor in the safe and effective use of these drugs. Your doctor is the best qualified person to advise you about a *prescription* drug for your individual use. . . .

Under Federal law, manufacturers of prescription drugs are required to give the medical profession full information on their products. The FDA has the authority to supervise the labeling and advertising of prescription drugs to assure that both are informative and accurate. On the recommendation of the Advisory Committee on Obstetrics and Gynecology, the FDA recently required uniform labeling for all the oral contraceptives so that the labeling for each drug provides information about experiences with the entire class of drugs, as well as with the particular product.

The Advisory Committee reviewed all of the available information regarding the usefulness and the risks which may be associated with the oral contraceptives. The Committee found "no adequate scientific data at this time proving these compounds unsafe for human use." The Committee did point out significant unanswered questions about the effects of oral contraceptives and urged research to obtain these answers. The FDA and other Federal agencies have undertaken a number of research projects to meet this need for additional data.

New and different drugs for conception control are now under investigation by scientists and physicians in various academic institutions and in industry. Under Federal law, the FDA monitors all investigations in which experimental drugs are used in humans.

However, information on investigational drugs is submitted to the FDA on a confidential basis. When the scientific evidence gathered from these investigations establishes the safety and effectiveness of a new drug, the drug is approved for marketing.

October 25, 1969.

Kathryn wrote a letter to Robert H. Finch, Secretary of the Department of Health, Education and Welfare. She knew that oral contraceptives violated the Federal Food, Drug and Cosmetic Act.

I am a doctoral candidate at Harvard University with a double major in Public Law and Government and International Law.

I have written numerous letters to officials other than yourself—Dr. Ley of the FDA for example—without the courtesy of a response. I have read that you are a progressive, fair-minded, dedicated civil servant, and I hope that this letter will be given your consideration. I expect an answer.

What prompted my writing to you was a page one article in *The New York Times* today reporting your decision to ban cyclamates.

Bravo!!! Even though the sugar industry certainly isn't going to compel President Nixon to make you change your decision. But now that cyclamates are being attacked, how about birth control pills?

From my reading of *The New York Times* there is as much condemning evidence that the hormones in The Pill have caused illnesses as there is in the animal experiments showing unfavorable side effects from cyclamates. Look, I have had a run-in with the American Cancer Society on this subject and I know of the repressive tactics being used by the AMA so I realize this is a politically touchy subject. But so help me, I know that the birth control pills can be dangerous! I also know that there are too many interest groups in this country who don't care about a few deaths or deformities as long as they can peddle their product. What we need is a high public-minded official who does care and who is not afraid to at least label these pills as "possibly hazardous to your health."

I have researched this subject and I know that there is at the very least an enormous amount of doubt concerning the safety of these pills and yet physicians recommend them on the false premise that they are "perfectly safe."

Mr. Secretary, I would be most anxious to confer with you on this in the event you are not aware of the data pointing to their potential danger. A doctor at the American Cancer Society admitted to me that The Pill was really regarded as still experimental (in fact he advised his daughters not to take it for health reasons) but he nevertheless insisted that as far as the public ought to know, it is the best thing going.

When I disagreed, he told me to stop worrying about the millions of women who are presently taking The Pill and just start worrying about my own condition since I am a likely candidate for reoccurrence of breast cancer at age twenty-two.

This kind of scare tactic is obviously a pitiful substitute for logical discussion, resorted to by desperate people because there is in fact no intelligent excuse for presenting this lie to the public.

I intend to get to the bottom of this situation and I am most anxious to learn how you feel about The Pill and where you stand. I will await a response from you. Thank you for your consideration.

Respectfully yours,
Kathryn Stuart Huffman

Kathryn's letter to Secretary Finch was never acknowledged. On October 29, 1969, she wrote to Representative James J. Delaney:

> I am writing to you because I have just learned that you have been extremely active and diligent in making the long overdue ban on cyclamates possible. I was particularly interested in learning that this was done through your amendment to the 1938 Food, Drug and Cosmetic Act which prohibits the use of chemicals in foods if they have been found to cause cancer in humans or animals.
>
> Sir, I feel that I am presently working on an issue very much related to yours: the prohibition of chemicals in drugs which have been found to cause cancer in humans or animals.
>
> For the last nineteen months, since I began taking birth control pills and subsequently developed breast cancer at the age of twenty-two, I have been researching the issue of the safety of birth control pills in general, and their relation to cancer in particular.
>
> I have found that, as in the case of cyclamates, there are many interest groups sponsoring The Pill: the drug industry, the AMA, the Planned Parenthood Federation, and so on. On the other hand, I believe I have also found some interesting facts about these pills which indicate a need for their suppression if not their complete extinction.
>
> There is no question that the estrogen hormones in birth control pills will, if given in sufficient quantities, cause tumors in animals that may be cancerous. The 1966 FDA Report on Oral Contraceptives says, "There is experimental evidence that estrogens closely related to those used in the oral contraceptives currently marketed will, when continuously given to dogs and other

animals, produce breast carcinoma.'' In the light of this evidence, Sir, would it not seem but logical to extend your amendment to cover birth control pills and other drugs?

I know from my reading and personal experience that many physicians falsely present The Pill and recommend it to even doubtful patients as being the best form of birth control possible. The fact is, Congressman, they simply have no idea as to how safe The Pill is because it is still in the experimental stage. In most cases there is no information distributed to Pill users by either physicians or pharmacists about possible counterindications.

From the *Times* article it would appear that you've gone through Hell to get a sensible piece of legislation passed, and I can understand why you might prefer not to take on the drug manufacturers, the AMA, the Planned Parenthood Federation and the general public clamor for this expedient form of birth control. But as long as the status quo persists, many women are taking these pills and are going to go through the Hell of suffering from the resultant side effects—blood clots, blindness, paralysis and cancer, to name just a few.

I have been in contact with a number of people. So far I have received sympathetic replies saying that it is too soon to act, unsympathetic replies telling me to mind my own business, and no replies at all. I want to find an avenue for action. I want to see something done soon, because every day that passes will be another day in which millions of women, women who have ·been deluded by our government, will be poisoning themselves with these pills of undetermined risk. I sincerely hope that you are interested in attacking this situation and I anxiously await hearing your position on it.

Thank you for having taken an unpopular stand on an

issue for the benefit of the American public; thank you for reading this letter and giving consideration to another plea for the public welfare.

Very truly yours,
Kathryn Stuart Huffman

Congressman Delaney responded to Kathryn's letter sharing his concern with her regarding the potential dangers of The Pill. About six weeks later, Kathryn read an article by Victor Cohn, in *The Washington Post*. It indicated that some impact was being felt in Washington.

Dr. Herbert L. Ley, Jr., until three weeks ago Food and Drug Administration commissioner, says the government must consider action to see that the 8.5 million American women taking birth control pills get much greater information of their possible ill effects.

In fact, he said in an interview, they should be given much the same facts doctors get, in plain language—perhaps in a printed insert in every oral contraceptive package.

This could mean giving women several hundred words of information on how the pills sometimes cause blood clots, strokes and skin discoloration, and how they may be involved in liver, thyroid, urinary and vaginal problems; changes in pituitary, ovarian, and other hormone functions; eye trouble; depression and suicidal urges.

This view represents an important switch for Dr. Ley. Only last October, asked whether women shouldn't be given more information, he said he believed sufficient medical supervision is exercised.

*Victor Cohn, *The Washington Post*.

Dr. Ley left the Department of Health, Education and Welfare when he was relieved of his job and offered a so-called "promotion."

Now, he said, "Speaking as a private citizen and as a concerned physician, I feel a need for greater information for the patient. This is triggered in part by the fracas in Britain this month."

This was a surprising announcement by the British government's Committee on Safety of Drugs urging Pill makers and doctors to stop dispensing heavy dose oral contraceptives—21 of 30 brands—for fear of blood clots and other effects.

Also, Dr. Ley said, his new feeling is the crystallization of his thinking about the whole category of drugs to prevent something, given to healthy people—compounds like birth control pills, cholesterol drugs and preventive vaccines, all of which sometimes have undesirable effects.

"It is a feeling," he explained, "that giving drugs to the healthy is a whole different football game from giving drugs to a patient with acute pneumonia."

At the moment Congress recognizes only prescription and over-the-counter-drugs, so the idea that some prescription drugs need to be accompanied by more information and patient choice would require recognition by statute of still another category.

A great many physicians are giving their patients adequate information about the birth control pill, he maintained. "I fear—though I have no proof—that some may not be and that is the reason for my concern," he added.

Much the same charge will be made later today in an announcement by Senator Gaylord Nelson, D-Wisconsin, that on January 14 his Senate monopoly subcommittee will begin hearings to learn whether women are being adequately informed of The Pill's known hazards.

"It appears evident," Nelson charges, "that a substantial number are not advised of any of the health hazards or side effects."

Nelson also states that:

● The package insert which drug firms must include in their shipments to druggists warns of many serious adverse effects associated with The Pill. But neither patients nor doctors commonly see it.

● Pamphlets prepared by the manufacturers and distributed directly to patients through physicians make light of the minor dangers and do not even mention the major dangers.

● Thousands of college girls are being subjected to Pill propaganda by a merely lukewarm warning on ill effects found in a text widely used by college students.

During the months from January to March, Kathryn went to Washington to attend the Senate hearings conducted by Senator Nelson. She was familiar with the vested interest that some members of Congress had in the industry, so she wasn't as shocked as some others appeared to be at the hostile cross-examination of some expert witnesses. Money talks, she realized. If she wanted action, she'd have to initiate it herself. And how better than to hit the drug firms in the pocketbook?

Kathryn resolved to begin a lawsuit against the two companies that made the birth control pills she had taken.

Kathryn's lawsuit was one of the early ones. One year later, Ralph Nader warned the American Medical Association that a rise in the number of malpractice and negligence suits was inevitable. The lack of internal control by the medical profession permitted the practice of inferior medicine. Sooner or later the public would strike back.

An article in *The New York Times* of November 9, 1970,

reported the charge by associates of Ralph Nader that the doctors had no uniform, enforced standards of quality, that weak efforts to police the doctors by the doctors themselves were useless, and that the public's only recourse was the malpractice suit. But that could only be used after the damage was done.

May 1, 1970.

Kathryn went to New York and met with Paul Slater, the attorney who specialized in malpractice suits.

They had a long talk. They reviewed in detail the scientific information Kathryn had acquired since she took the first step of asking the family pharmacist for literature on The Pill. They discussed the medical aspects of her own case. Slater said her case justified a lawsuit. However, she also had to sue the two physicians who prescribed The Pill; the pharmaceutical companies would place the blame on her doctors for misrepresenting The Pill to her as a "safe" drug.

July 23, 1970.

Michael Jefferson, who also specialized in malpractice suits, was retained to work with Paul Slater on Kathryn's case. Jefferson had his offices in New Jersey, the state where both the physicians and the pharmaceutical companies' head offices were located.

What follows is the legal record of Kathryn Stuart Huffman's fight to spare other women the tragedy she suffered. It is the record of the legal proceedings that ended in a court settlement—one of the first birth-control-pill/breast cancer cases to be settled in court.

The victory came too late for Kathryn herself—but it was her triumph, nevertheless.

Part Two

"The American woman, both rich and poor, black and white, is being victimized by social engineers. Population control rather than the health of the individual has become the new directing force of the family planning movement. . . .

"When preoccupation is with control rather than planning, people are viewed numerically as statistics, and concern for the welfare of the individual, the person, diminishes. An effective contraceptive rather than a safe one becomes prime consideration and the technological achievement replaces the humanistic goal. . . . Despite the fact that we knew in advance that a powerful chemical disruptive of normal physiological mechanisms was being introduced, The Pill has been the most poorly tested drug ever approved by the FDA. . . .

"Although many other drugs have been removed from the market for lesser reasons, we must wonder why The Pill has been retained despite the massive accumulation of medical hazards and metabolic disturbances reported from clinical medicine and laboratories. . . . The population control experts, in promoting The Pill regardless of safety are practicing chemical warfare on the women of this country. . . ."

> Herbert Ratner, M.D.
> Editor, Child & Family Quarterly
> The Medical Hazards of the Birth Control Pill
> *Child and Family Reprint Booklet*
> Oak Park, Illinois 1969

Chapter One

October 12, 1970.

Kathryn received a letter from her lawyer, Mike Jefferson:

Thank you for sending me the details of your medical condition. I know it must have been painful for you to describe your illness in such depth. I also want to thank you for the excellent way you answered the interrogatories [written questions].

The next step will be the taking of your deposition, scheduled for October 24th. As you know, the deposition is actually a question-and-answer session between you and the lawyers for the drug companies and the doctors named in your suit.

Everything you say will be recorded by a court reporter. This then becomes your testimony, under oath, and may be referred to when your case comes to trial. Of course, there is no judge or referee at the deposition. Objections and motions will be made by lawyers during the deposition. They become a matter of record for the judge to review at a later date. If a serious objection results in an impasse, we may have to postpone the deposition until the matter is reviewed by a judge.

There are several reasons for taking the deposition. I guess the major reason is to give the defendants' lawyers a chance to explore issues with you so they can be better prepared for the trial. They also want to minimize surprises. Often the deposition leads to an out-of-court settlement. You have already refused several substantial offers from the defendants to settle. They probably will approach you again after the deposition.

I doubt that the doctors you are suing will attend your deposition. We will take their depositions after yours is completed. You may want to attend theirs.

Paul and I have been working on the brief in your case. To date, the charge is that a non-active, pre-existing cancer was stimulated to grow into a palpable lump in your breast as the result of your use of two oral contraceptive pills made by the defendants. As a result of your breast cancer, your breast was removed. Nevertheless, the cancer spread, and your life is now in danger.

The drug manufacturers are also charged with failure to exercise due care in the development of The Pill, failure to adequately test The Pill, and failure to adequately warn of the dangerous side effects of The Pill. The evidence will show that there was no warning accompanying the product for you to read. You had to rely on the prescribing doctors to share information with you about The Pill.

The prescribing doctors are being charged with negligence. It was improper for them to give you false reassurances of safety in recommending The Pill. Since there are many ways of preventing pregnancy, you should have been given a choice. The choice should be made by the woman (not her doctor or her husband) whose body alone is involved. This choice must be based upon the full information available. Your doctors failed to share that information with you. Furthermore, your doctors failed to disclose to you any information about the risk of The Pill in stimulating breast cancer. This scientific knowledge goes back many years and they should have been alert to this possibility.

Attached are the guidelines I give my clients before they go to trial. You might find them helpful to review before the deposition.

Guidelines For Witnesses

1. *Tell the truth*—a lie may lose the case. In a law suit (as in other matters) honesty is the best policy.

Telling the truth, however, means more than refraining from telling a deliberate falsehood. Telling the truth requires that a witness testify accurately about what he knows. If you tell the truth and tell it accurately, you have nothing to fear on cross-examination.

2. *Don't guess*—if you don't know, say you don't know.

3. Be sure that you *understand the question* before you attempt to give an answer. You can't possibly give a truthful and accurate answer unless you understand the question. If necessary, ask the lawyer to repeat it. He will probably ask the court reporter to read it back.

4. *Take your time*—give the question such thought as it requires to understand it and formulate your answer, and then give the answer.

5. *Answer the question* that is asked and then stop. Don't volunteer information.

6. Talk loud enough so everybody can hear you. Don't chew gum; keep your hands away from your mouth. You can't speak distinctly while chewing gum or with your hand over your mouth.

7. Give an audible answer so the court reporter can get it. Don't nod your head yes or no.

8. Don't look at the lawyer for help when you're on the stand. You're on your own. You won't get any help from the judge either. If you look at your lawyer when a question is asked on cross-examination, or for his approval after answering a question, the jury is bound to notice it and it will create a bad impression.

9. Beware of questions involving distances and time. If you make an estimate, make sure that everyone understands that you are estimating.

10. Know your name, where you live, how old you are, and when you were married, etc.

11. Don't fence or argue with the lawyer on the other

side. He has a right to question you, and if you give him impertinent or evasive answers you may be reprimanded by the judge.

12. Don't lose your temper no matter how hard you are pressed. Lose your temper and you may lose the case. If you lose your temper, you have played right into the hands of the cross-examiner.

13. Be courteous. Being courteous is one of the best ways to make a good impression on the court and jury. Don't be afraid to answer "Yes, sir" and "No, sir" and to address the judge as "Your Honor."

14. If asked whether you have talked to the lawyer on your side, or to an investigator, admit it freely.

15. Avoid joking and wisecracks. A lawsuit is a serious matter.

16. Don't be afraid to look the jury in the eye and tell the story. Jurors are naturally sympathetic to the witness and want to hear what he has to say.

17. Give a positive answer when you can. Don't let the lawyer on the other side catch you by asking whether you are willing to swear to your version of what you know because you saw or heard it. If you were there and know what happened or didn't happen, don't be afraid to "swear" to it. You were "sworn" to tell the truth when you took the stand.

18. Steer clear of jurors during recesses. Under no circumstances should you approach a juror, even concerning a matter wholly foreign to the case on trial. To do so is to invite suspicion.

Chapter Two

October 24, 1970, 12:10 P.M.

The deposition of Kathryn Stuart Huffman began in the law office of Michael Jefferson. The office was in a large modern building in the midst of an eroded neighborhood in downtown Newark.

Kathryn sat with her mother and Mike Jefferson at the smaller of two tables in the firm's conference room. Facing them from across the room at the other table were twelve men—lawyers representing the four defendants. Each of the defendants, the two doctors and two pharmaceutical companies, had lawyers from a different firm. The court reporter sat to the side, between the two tables.

Kathryn felt twelve pairs of eyes on her. She looked steadily over at the other table and watched the men as they sat, talking in low voices.

Kathryn was the David to this collective Goliath. Only five foot two, weighing 105 pounds, she looked fully ready to fight. The set of her small chin belied the soft grace of her features. She wore a brown suede jumper over a beige silk shirt. Her left hand and arm, wrapped in an elastic bandage, rested in a brown silk scarf made into a sling. A sheaf of papers lay on the table in front of her.

To Kathryn's left sat Mike, a man in his forties with graying black hair and hazel eyes. He had the reputation of only taking cases to trial that he knew he could win. Mike spoke well extemporaneously, backed up by the extensive research he undertook before every proceeding he was involved in. A man of great charm and appeal, he made a romantic figure in court.

Mike's goals were idealistic. He worked toward his vision of a better world. He was a leader in the World Federalist movement. Mike and Kathryn had a mutual interest. They shared the same ideals and spoke the same language.

The court reporter opened the session: "Kathryn Stuart Huffman, the plaintiff, having been duly sworn, begins her testimony. Direct examination by Mr. John H. Baylor, representing the Roth Pharmaceutical Company, defendant."

Baylor rose, turned to Kathryn, and began a lawsuit that made history.

"Mrs. Huffman, I am John H. Baylor, the attorney for the Roth Pharmaceutical Company, manufacturer of Cyclemide, the first birth control pill you took. I want to remind you that you have previously been duly sworn according to law by the notary public and court reporter who is recording this deposition." Baylor's appearance was disarming, a casual, country-style lawyer around sixty who looked as though he would rather be fishing or playing golf right then. He had a flat, monotonous voice.

"Mrs. Huffman, this is a deposition," he continued. "We are going to ask you a number of questions about the case that you have filed here against the Roth Pharmaceutical Corporation, the Lears Pharmaceutical Corporation, Dr. Benedict Lawrence and Dr. Vittorio Canaris. If there is any question that you do not understand, will you advise us of that fact?"

"Yes, I will."

"Everything you say is being taken down by the court reporter."

"I understand."

"And if you answer something without really understanding it, you may make a mistake. We do not want you to do that, not only for your sake but for our sake. If there is some question that causes complete confusion, if you want to ask us off the record, I will personally have no objection. Indicate that and we will explain it to you. All right?"

"Yes."

"Your name is Mrs. Kathryn Stuart Huffman?"

"That is correct."

"How old are you?"

"Twenty-four years old."

"When were you married?"

"June 23, 1968."

"Where?"

"At the Waldorf in New York City."

"What is the name of your husband?"

"Dr. Conrad Huffman."

"What kind of a doctor is he?"

"He's a physician."

There followed a series of questions, establishing that Kathryn was born in San Antonio, Texas, on November 7, 1945, that her mother was twenty-two at the time and forty-seven currently, and that as far as Kathryn knew, her mother had never been pregnant except with Kathryn herself.

Baylor paused, formulating his next question. With a change of expression, he glared at Kathryn, and went on: "Now, you allege that on or about April 11, 1968, you employed Dr. Benedict Lawrence to examine you and prescribe a plan for you to prevent pregnancy. This was while your husband was completing his medical training. Did you see the doctor for that purpose?"

"Yes."

"Who was present at the time you had this first conversation with Dr. Lawrence?"

"Just Dr. Lawrence and myself. I told him that I was getting married, and that I had discussed birth control with my future husband, and he was very anxious for me to take the birth control pill but I had doubts about it. I wanted his opinion."

"When you went to see him you wanted his advice on what to use?"

"Yes. I left it wide open. I'd have been extremely happy for him to say, 'I think your husband should use a condom.' I didn't tell him not to say that. I just asked him for his advice about birth control measures because I had doubts about The Pill. He said I should take The Pill—that was his opinion."

"Tell us what he said, please."

"He said you take something like seven pills for four weeks, and then you have your period, and then you wait a week and take them again. He said the directions would be on The Pill container so I wouldn't have to worry about it.

"I might say I was very surprised that he wanted me to take The Pill, because he had told my mother not to take it. I really didn't want to take The Pill. Just the idea of interfering with the normal menstrual cycle seemed to me to be a bad idea. But he said it was a *good* idea and I had to rely on his opinion."

"Did he say it was a good idea or did he just answer your questions? Did he say 'it's the best form or safest form of contraceptive'?"

"He said it was the safest, and also a good idea."

"Did he say it was a good idea?"

"Well. . . ."

"If you can remember," Mike Jefferson cautioned Kathryn.

"I believe he said something to that effect."

"You are not telling us now you remember him saying it is a good idea, but that you think it was something to that effect?"

"Yes. He has a very casual way of talking."

"Had you communicated with your husband that you did not want to take these pills?"

"Yes. We had a discussion about that. But I felt I was kind of contributing to the marriage by going along with what my husband wanted to do if my doctor agreed. Furthermore, my husband was a resident doctor at that time. I felt the only way I could refute his argument was to have a medical person, you know, a physician back me up, and Dr. Lawrence didn't do that."

"Dr. Lawrence, what?"

"He didn't do that. He more went along with my husband's way of thinking in saying The Pill was safe and that he would recommend it."

"Did you tell Dr. Lawrence that you did not want to take it?"

"Yes, I told him that I was apprehensive about taking it. He told me my concern was not well founded."

"Did you tell him that you did *not* want to take The Pill? That is my question!"

"I would say—I told him I wanted his advice."

Baylor removed his glasses and shook them at her. Angrily, he asked, "Will you answer my question? Did you tell the doctor that you did not want to take contraceptive pills?"

Mike Jefferson motioned to Kathryn to remain silent. "I am going to have to interrupt and suggest that you are arguing with the witness. She has answered your two previous questions in the best way she could. In effect, if you want a negative answer, it's in the record. She did not say, 'I don't want to take The Pill.' What she did say is what she has repeated three times. I think you are badgering the witness. I would suggest it is unnecessary."

"First of all," Baylor said as he frowned at Mike, "I don't badger young ladies. I am entitled to an answer to my question. I press the question because she has not answered one way or the other. You may infer it one way or the other, but I don't prefer to infer. I want an answer. I would like an answer to the question."

Mike Jefferson looked at Kathryn. "Let me instruct the witness. Mrs. Huffman, counsel is entitled to a direct answer and if he gives you a direct question, try to give him first at least a direct answer, and then you may explain it. This way we won't get tied up. Do you understand?"

Kathryn took a sip of water, then looked at the defense attorney.

"I would say I told him that I was apprehensive about taking The Pill and that I would leave it up to his good judgment to tell me one way or the other."

"How old were you at that time? Were you twenty-three? You were born in 1945. We are talking about 1968."

"I was twenty-two."

"You were twenty-two years old?"

"Yes."

"Had you graduated already from Wellesley at the time of this conversation?"

"Yes."

"Had you at any time, in the course of your studies, studied any course in physiology?"

"No."

"Had you had any hygiene courses in college or anyplace else?"

"Not in that field—in biology, yes."

"Had you read up on anything at all about the question of contraceptives before you saw Dr. Lawrence?"

"A friend had brought over an article in a popular magazine about The Pill."

"Had you read the information?"

"Yes."

"Had you discussed that information with your husband?"

"Yes. He told me, as a resident physician, that the article was a lot of baloney."

"What was this article? Do you remember that?"

"I believe it was in *Good Housekeeping.*"

"What other articles did you read on the subject before you saw Dr. Lawrence?"

"That is the only one I can remember."

"Did Dr. Lawrence say anything else to you at the first meeting about using The Pill?"

"Yes. He told me that he would recommend that I use it as soon as possible because I could expect some unpleasantness, that I could expect unpleasant side effects from The Pill such as nausea and headaches and that my body had to become accustomed to these feelings. He said it would be a good idea if I could get over those unpleasant side effects before I got married so I could enjoy my honeymoon.''

"Nausea and what?''

"Headaches.''

"Did he discuss any other possible side effects from the use of the contraceptive?''

"No, just nausea and the headaches and maybe sore breasts. The nausea and headaches stuck in my mind.''

"We are still talking about April 11th?''

"Yes.''

"He said to start using it, so you could enjoy your honeymoon?'' Baylor repeated. "Was he discussing a particular kind of contraceptive pill?''

"No, it was very general.''

"Did he make any recommendation during this April 11th visit of any particular pill?''

"He said, 'I would like you to start with Cyclemide.' ''

"And see how it works?''

"Yes.''

"What does that mean to you?''

"I really don't know.''

"Didn't you ask him what he meant by that?''

"I think he said the side effects would last for about three months, and if they did not go away I could try something else. I'm sure of that. He said for three months the side effects would continue to decrease. If not, I could try another pill. He told me that not every pill would agree with me,'' she explained. "This business about the side effects, and so on. It was given a three-month trial period.''

"He told you he wanted you to take Cyclemide three months and the side effects would probably be over by then, and then take another pill?''

"No. If the side effects did not occur, or if they decreased, I assumed he would have kept me on Cyclemide."

"When did you begin to take Cyclemide?"

"I can't remember the exact date, but I believe I started in April, at the latest."

"You got a prescription for it?"

"Yes, I got a prescription for it."

"Where did you have it filled?"

"Van's Pharmacy, in Short Hills, New Jersey." Kathryn consulted the papers before her on the table.

"Did you have this prescription for Cyclemide renewed on any occasion?"

"I think that there were about three cycles in it, so I don't believe I had any occasion to have it renewed."

"Now, in referring to The Pill, what do you mean by 'safe?' "

"I didn't want to get sick or die from it."

"Did Dr. Lawrence tell you it was safe?"

"Yes."

"Did he use those words?"

"Yes, that it was 'safe.' "

"He also told you that you would have side effects."

"Yes, he did."

"And the side effects made you sick, didn't they?"

"Well, not what I would call 'sick,' " she answered, " 'Sick' is when you have to call a doctor and say, 'Please come over, I am sick.' Unpleasant, uncomfortable, that's the way the side effects seemed to make me feel."

"Before you went to see Dr. Lawrence on April 11, did you discuss with your mother and/or your father this problem of whether or not you would take The Pill?"

"Yes. My mother was against it. She is sort of against pills in general—you know, anything that would disturb the natural function of the body. That's why, I guess, her friend, Olga Johnson, thought she'd want to see the article in *Good Housekeeping* about The Pill."

"When did you get engaged to be married?"

"Around November of 1966."

"When did you start the discussions with either your prospective husband, your mother or father about this idea of taking some kind of pill to prevent pregnancy?"

"I don't believe it was until April of 1968."

"At that time had your wedding date been set?"

"Yes."

"When did you have your first discussion with your mother about this?"

"I suppose it was in April."

"Was it before you went to Dr. Lawrence or after?"

"Before."

"What did you say and what did she say?"

"I said, 'Conrad wants me to use birth control pills.' She said, 'That's not such a good idea.' We discussed this article. I said I'd have to get a doctor's opinion because Conrad would only accept something a physician said."

"What did your mother have to say about this, other than the fact she was against it?"

"She said, 'Great, see Dr. Lawrence.' She felt he would give me the same advice that he had given her. She was upset when I came home and said that Dr. Lawrence had prescribed The Pill."

"Did you read any of the literature that came with the Cyclemide pills when you got them?"

"The only literature that came with the Cyclemide when I got them was a little sheet with directions about when to take them."

"Did Dr. Lawrence say the only side effects would be nausea and headaches and sometimes sore breasts? Is that the only warning that you say he gave you about taking The Pill?"

"Yes, and right about the time that I was beginning to take The Pill, there was an article in *The New York Times* about thrombophlebitis and The Pill. A report from England said there were signs of a relationship. I called the doctor and asked him about this. He rejected it out of hand. He said, 'Absolutely insignificant,' and gave me some argument about the chances of my dying during pregnancy outweighing that. . . ."

Baylor cut her off. "Were you afraid you might die in pregnancy?"

"No. I was young and healthy. Conrad and I were looking forward to having children. We'd already picked out names for our children." Kathryn paused. She looked down at some papers on the table to hide the tears that filled her eyes. Within seconds she seemed to regain control. "Recently I read a book by Morton Mintz. He says doctors often use this argument about the risk of dying during pregnancy. Mintz explains that The Pill induces a false state of pregnancy every month. There is no fetus or embryonic tissue to protect the mother's body from hormones that can cause cancer."

"What's the name of the book Mintz wrote?"

"*The Pill—An Alarming Report*."

"When did it come out?"

"1969. A year after I started to take The Pill," she added.

Chapter Three

Later the same day, October 24, 1970.

Baylor resumed his questioning.

"Did you discuss with your father the prospect of your taking The Pill?"

"No. My father was lecturing in Europe around that time."

"Now, did your mother say anything further to you about taking The Pill before you started to take it?"

"I think she was trying to be a very good mother-in-law. She had a very definite opinion that I shouldn't take The Pill, but she was being put down by medical opinion and couldn't press it."

"In this article that you read in *Good Housekeeping*, did that talk about side effects?"

"It mentioned the fact that The Pill was kind of new on the market, that they didn't know much about it, and it was kind of experimental, which scared me."

"Did you say to the doctor that you were scared of it, that it was experimental and they did not know too much about it?"

"I don't know if I said it in those words. I said I was apprehensive about taking The Pill."

"I see. What I am trying to find out is, you were apprehensive. You were apprehensive about what?"

"The fact that The Pill was new, and that it was in fact experimental to a certain extent. They didn't know much about it. Then this report coming out when I started taking The Pill, from England, saying they found blood clotting. If they found that—," Kathryn paused, then made her point, "they could have found other things as time went on."

"Did you discuss this apprehension with your husband?"

"Yes. He said he learned in medical school it was perfectly safe. He said he discussed The Pill with his professors and colleagues and there was no foundation for my apprehension."

"Did you accept his advice that it was perfectly safe then?"

Kathryn sensed a trap. "I really didn't accept his advice. He was inexperienced in medicine. It was the advice of Dr. Lawrence that I accepted."

"When this thing came out in the paper about England, did you read any more on the subject from anyplace else?"

"No."

"When you got Cyclemide, did it have the word Cyclemide on the box or carton?"

Kathryn, holding her right index finger and thumb about two inches apart, asked, "Do you mean one of those little containers?"

"I don't use them—I don't know," was the sarcastic reply.

Kathryn continued, "It's a kind of plastic container, a dispenser. It says, 'Cyclemide.' It gives directions about when to take the pills. It says nothing about side effects or anything."

"Didn't it have a little insert with it? You are shaking your head no? Didn't it have a little insert all folded up and little tiny writing talking about the history of it, the background of it, side effects, how to take it, and so forth? Wasn't that in there?"

"No. I'm certain it wasn't in there."

At Kathryn's response, Baylor scratched his head, let his glasses drop down on his nose, dramatizing his disbelief. There *must* have been an insert in the pill box container!

Kathryn went on, "If I had had the opportunity to read such an insert, I would never have taken The Pill, no matter what any doctor told me. As a matter of fact, I later got in touch with the FDA and some members of Congress to urge them to work for legislation making it compulsory that such information accompany The Pill—and other medication prescribed by physicians, too."

Baylor ignored Kathryn's comment and asked, "Did you ask Dr. Lawrence whether or not there was anything that you could read on the subject to help reassure you?"

"No. He appeared annoyed that I asked so many questions. I was weary of pursuing the whole thing by now, and I didn't like the hostility that it was causing between Conrad and myself. I just took Dr. Lawrence's word. He was trained in medicine and I wasn't."

"Did you take Cyclemide then for awhile?"

"Yes."

"Did you get any side effects?"

"Oh, yes," she responded.

"What were the side effects?"

Kathryn thought for a moment. "All that Dr. Lawrence said, I got. I got headaches, nausea, sore breasts, acne. I don't know if he mentioned acne."

"What is acne?"

"My skin was broken out a great deal—pimples."

"Did you tell him about that?"

"My mother called him and told him about her concern and mine regarding my side effects. He told her that I'd be okay and my body would get accustomed to The Pill. He told her to stop 'smothering' me and that he wanted me to stay on The Pill."

"Let me ask you this, when was the first time you had these headaches, nausea and soreness? How soon after you began to take The Pill did this occur?"

"I would say within two weeks at the latest."

"Weren't you concerned then?"

"As I said before, Dr. Lawrence told me to expect those side effects."

"Weren't you concerned, however, when you got acne, which according to you he had not mentioned?"

"No, because I had heard of other people who were having the same side effects and my mother discussed this matter of acne with him."

"Can you tell me why you did not go to Dr. Lawrence for your blood test when you were going to be married?"

"We were getting married in New York. It seemed convenient to do everything in New York."

"When your husband told you that as a resident physician he knew The Pill was okay, did you ask him what literature he had read, what information he had obtained about The Pill and its possible side effects?"

"Yes. He said he had learned it from his professors and colleagues."

"Did you ask him whether he had been reading any literature? This is my question!"

"I did. He said he obtained opinions at first hand from experts who practiced medicine."

"Didn't you in fact ask your husband whether or not you had to worry about anything like phlebitis and so forth yourself? Didn't you ask him that?"

"By that time he had gone back to California. He wasn't around. The answer to your question is no."

"Did you ever ask him that question even after you got married?"

"No. Once I started taking The Pill and experienced the bad side effects, it took a lot of determination on my part to see it through for the three-month period."

"Did you call your husband and tell him about all those side effects you were getting?"

"Yes, but he kept telling me my body would adjust to them."

Removing his eyeglasses and biting on one end of the earpiece, Baylor remarked, "You make these side effects seem severe."

"Well, they were pretty uncomfortable, but not as severe as the pain and discomfort I feel today," said Kathryn.

Baylor ignored the latter part of her answer. "Did your mother again advise you not to keep taking them?"

"No. Both Dr. Lawrence and my fiancé told her that her concern was unfounded, so she did not pursue the issue. She didn't want to alienate her future son-in-law or make matters worse for me."

"Did your mother have any influence upon your decisions up to the time when you were married?"

"I believe she had as much influence over me as most mothers have over their children. I respected my mother's opinions but I made my own decisions."

"As you have gotten older, reaching up to the point of your getting married, did you discuss all of the things that you would feel with your mother?"

"I discussed many things with my mother, but not *all* things."

"Did you take her advice on all occasions?"

"No. That's why I am here now . . . this was one of the times I didn't take her advice. She told me *not* to take The Pill."

"She said you should not take The Pill?"

"Yes."

"When did she tell you that?"

"That was in April of 1968 when my husband came home for the Easter vacation. We talked about what kind of contraceptive devices we could use. . . . I discussed it with my mother afterward, after I discussed it with him. She said, 'I don't want you to take The Pill because I heard there were serious problems associated with it.' There was nothing specific mentioned. She also said that her father, who was a pharmacist, had warned her about taking medication that went against nature. He had warned her about changing 'normal' metabolism and using hormones. She respected her father's opinion."

"Did you discuss The Pill with your mother's father?"

"No. He died in 1962."

"I think you told us you married in June of 1968?"

"Yes, June 23rd."

"Where did you go on your honeymoon?"

"We went to Europe."

"Where did you go and how long were you gone altogether?"

"We went to Copenhagen, Salzburg and Venice. We were gone about twelve days altogether. We had to cut our trip short as my husband had to take some examinations in New York two weeks after our wedding."

"Did you take your pills while you were in Europe every day?"

"The Cyclemide, yes. In fact, my husband asked me every day, 'Did you take The Pill?' "

"Did you discuss with your husband the fact you were not feeling well?"

"He was aware that I was unable to eat much because I was nauseated, my breasts were tender and sore, and I had constant headaches."

"That continued for how long?"

"It kept getting worse in June and July. By the end of July it seemed to be worse than when I started taking them. It didn't make any sense to me whatsoever."

"Could you describe these headaches for us?"

There were beads of perspiration on Kathryn's forehead. She patted her face with her handkerchief. "Mr. Baylor, I have had so much pain since then, I don't think I can describe the headaches."

"They were bad enough, however, that you knew they were with you every day at that time?"

"Yes."

"We are now talking about the end of July."

"Actually, it was the nausea that bothered me the most."

"Was that there all the time?"

"Just about all the time, I would say."

"Did these side effects continue up to August?"

"Yes, that's why I saw Dr. Canaris in August."

"Were you taking the Cyclemide up to the time you saw Dr. Canaris?"

"Yes. I went to Dr. Canaris hoping he would tell me to stop taking them so I could present my husband with a medical opinion."

"Why did you choose Dr. Canaris?"

"My grandmother and some friends of the family had been examined by him. He was a gynecologist and it seemed to me it was about time I saw a gynecologist."

"Wasn't Dr. Lawrence a gynecologist?"

"No, he's an internist."

"He never represented to you he was a gynecologist in any way?"

"No."

There was silence for a moment before the lawyer again took up the questioning. "Now, we're going to Dr. Canaris. All right?"

"Yes."

"When you conferred with him, did you confer with him alone or was someone else present?"

Kathryn shook her head. "Just the two of us."

"What did you tell him and what did he tell you?"

"I told him the side effects from the pills were really getting worse, that I was growing more apprehensive about taking them and could he please, as a gynecologist, tell me to get off those pills. I told him I needed his recommendation to discontinue using The Pill so I could tell my husband a doctor had advised me to do it. He told me he never had a patient who complained as much as I did about The Pill. That he felt the complaints were in my mind and I was imagining the side effects. He told me the birth control pills were the best form of contraceptive I could use and that he would do me a favor of sorts by putting me on Mordrine instead of Cyclemide. He felt if he changed the drug, I might feel better about it psychologically."

"You went to him hoping he would tell you to get off The Pill?"

"Yes, because my husband kept saying they were wonderful. Therefore, if I had a doctor who said he had some doubt about The Pill, then I could go to Conrad and say, 'This doctor thinks The Pill is harmful to me.' "

"You couldn't stop taking them yourself?"

"Not logically. To my husband it would have seemed as if I didn't have the courage to last it out or something. My husband was quite aggressive and persistent. Particularly when the subject had to do with medicine."

"Did Dr. Canaris examine you?"

"Yes, he did and I was pretty tense during the examination and he concluded I was neurotic."

"You are not telling us he concluded from the internal examination that you were neurotic?"

"He said, 'Are you frigid with your husband?' I said, 'Why do you ask me that?' He said, 'Well, you were terribly tense during the internal examination.' I said, 'What do you expect? This is one of my first internal examinations.' "

"*Were* you frigid with your husband?" Baylor asked.

"No. As a matter of fact, my husband bragged to others that I was quite good in bed."

Mike's annoyance at this line of questioning by Baylor was about even with Kathryn's and he decided not to remain silent any longer. "May I interrupt to note on the record that I think this is far afield. I am not going to instruct the witness not to answer the questions, but I will leave it to the discretion of the trial court on a later motion. I just cannot see how this material is relevant to this medical malpractice case or even relevant on the issue of credibility, but, Mr. Baylor, if you feel you want to continue the subject, you may do so over my objection."

Baylor replied, "I don't want to continue the subject. But I think in view of what the lady has said with respect to the reasons for her divorce, and so forth, that these may be very, very pertinent."

"Is it your understanding that in this case we are seeking money damages because of the divorce?" Mike asked.

"The case is too young for me to know what you're seeking. Therefore, I am attempting to take a deposition on all things that may lead to discovery of material which would be relevant in this case," Baylor replied.

"Let me state for the record," Mike continued, "that we are not seeking money damages for the divorce in this particular case or in any other case."

"I understand, Mr. Jefferson, since they are not as yet divorced, under the law of the State of New Jersey her present husband may very well be entitled to a cause of action for loss of services and/or consortium, even though he is not represented in this case at the present time. If he did file such a case, in my opinion, it would have legal validity—whether it would have factual efficacy is something entirely different."

"If you feel you should proceed on this line in order to protect yourself from later litigation, I am not terribly sympathetic to that approach in this case, but I will permit the witness to answer your questions, Mr. Baylor."

Baylor returned his attention to Kathryn. "What were the problems that were going on up to this time between you and your husband? Wasn't the biggest problem about this birth control pill?"

"That was one of them, yes."

"Wasn't that the biggest one?"

"I guess so."

"Isn't it a fact that you wanted to stop taking those pills?"

"Yes, but then I never wanted to take them in the first place."

Kathryn's reply obviously annoyed Baylor. "Did your husband recommend that you should use an IUD [intra-uterine device]?"

"No, he thought The Pill was still good. He had taken a position on that. The only people he feels are important are doctors. If I could say 'Dr. So-and-So' said The Pill is not good for me or that I shouldn't take it, my husband would consider changing his position."

"Did you tell Dr. Canaris you were married to a gentleman who was a physician?"

"No."

"Did you tell Dr. Canaris that you wanted to get off The Pill?"

"Yes, I did."

"Now, Mrs. Huffman, when you said to him, 'I want to get off The Pill' didn't he tell you if you wanted to get off, all you had to do was stop?"

Kathryn answered calmly, "No. He said it would be his advice for me to keep on taking it. I was relying on my doctor—he was the expert. He's the one who is supposed to give me medical supervision. He's the one who was given confidential information by the FDA, the drug firms and professional journals. I was given nothing to go by—only his comments that I was imagining the whole thing!"

Baylor frowned at Kathryn. "What did Dr. Canaris say to you when you described those side effects you were experiencing?"

"He said I was imagining them, that all my complaints were in my head. He said he never had a patient who complained as much as I did about The Pill. He concluded I was a neurotic female and there was no medical basis for my complaints about The Pill."

"The reason you kept taking The Pill was because of your husband's attitude. Is that right?"

"And the attitude of the medical profession that sustained his," Kathryn quickly added.

"What do you mean by 'the medical profession?' You only saw two doctors."

"I did the best I could," she replied. "Both physicians had been recommended to me by my family and friends. Both were trustees in highly reputable hospitals."

"Did you read anything during the time you were in Europe?"

"About The Pill? No, nothing."

"When you came back and you still had the side effects, did you read anything?"

"No."

"Have you read a lot since?"

"Yes. But I didn't read anything before I had the radical mastectomy."

"Since you became ill, did you ever read a package insert of Cyclemide?"

"Yes."

"Did you ever read a packet insert of Mordrine?"

"Yes. I went to the druggist and asked for one. He said one insert came in a carton, with several dozen packages of birth control pill containers. Dozens of containers were in a carton, but only one insert."

"You said there was only one insert for dozens of packages of birth control pill containers?" He had repeated the words 'dozens of packages.' It was evident that her reference to the one insert bothered him.

She reinforced what she had said. "Yes. They were packaged, say, dozens in a carton. There was one insert for the druggist. That is what the whole thing is with the Federal Drug Administration. That is why I went to Washington, wrote to Congressmen, went to Senate hearings and wrote to the FDA. If I had read the insert citing the contraindications and warnings concerning the birth control pill before I started taking it, I would have known that the doctors were misrepresenting the facts to me when they said The Pill would not jeopardize my health and said it was safe for me to take. They had only one insert and that was for the druggist. That is why I am here today."

"The whole thing is they do not have printed inserts with each package the customer buys, but just for the druggist to have?" Baylor was obviously trying to find a way to put this information he considered damning into some perspective.

"Yes," Kathryn replied. "Just this month I read an article that the Food and Drug Administration abandoned their plan to place warnings on all oral contraceptive packages because the drug manufacturers and the American Medical Association objected. The article quoted the doctors as saying that such literature would be considered an intrusion into the practice of medicine.''

"What was the title of this article?''

"I can get it for you later. It was in a journal for druggists. I have done a great deal of research since my radical mastectomy,'' Kathryn continued. "I started with the druggist. As soon after my surgery as I was able to get into a car, I asked my mother to drive me to the drugstore. I wanted to talk to the druggist to see if there was any information about The Pill. I felt The Pill was responsible for my breast cancer.''

"You're referring to your first operation—the radical mastectomy?''

"Yes. Before the surgery I was fearful of what might happen, but I hadn't tried to find out about the subject for myself. Again, I was depending on the doctors. After the radical mastectomy, I knew I couldn't rely completely on doctors anymore.''

"Now, was Mordrine ever prescribed for you?''

"Yes.''

"When did you get that?''

"The same day that I saw Dr. Canaris. He gave me a prescription for it and I started using it.''

"Did Dr. Canaris examine your breasts on that occasion?''

"Yes, he did a thorough examination.''

"Did he tell you whether or not he found anything in your breasts?''

"He said I was absolutely fine in every way except that he had to wait to see how the Pap test would turn out. [The Pap test is a cell test for indications of cancer in the female genitalia.] He said I was healthy.''

"What was the result of the Pap test?''

"It was negative.''

"Did you begin to take Mordrine?''

"Yes, that very day.''

"What color were they?''

"I think they were yellow tablets."

Mr. Baylor peered over his glasses at his young opponent. "All yellow?"

"Yes."

"Was there any printed insert in that package?"

"There were only directions telling you how to use The Pill, the same as with the Cyclemide, the same idea."

"Nothing else besides that?"

"No, nothing else."

"When you went to see," the lawyer glanced at his notes to get a name, "Mr. Logan, the druggist, on November 30 of 1968, did you ask him whether or not the Mordrine had inserts?"

"Yes, I asked him about both. He said, 'No. The druggist only gets one insert for all the packets.' "

"You are telling us Mr. Logan said in the case of both Cyclemide and Mordrine he only got one insert for a number of separate packages?"

"Yes, that's correct."

"Did you read that insert after November 30, 1968?"

"Yes, I certainly did," Kathryn replied with heat. She found a paper from among those on the table in front of her. "Here's what it says. 'The following adverse reactions have been observed with varying incidence in patients receiving oral contraceptives: Nausea, Vomiting, Gastrointestinal symptoms (such as abdominal cramps and bloating), Breakthrough bleeding, Spotting, Change in menstrual flow, Breast changes (tenderness, enlargement and secretion), Edema, Chloasma or melasma—' " Kathryn broke off. "Edema is fluid accumulation and swelling. Chloasma and melasma are skin discoloration."

She turned back to the printed sheet. " 'Cholestatic jaundice, Migraine, Rash (allergic), Mental depression, Change in weight (increase or decrease), Amenorrhea.' "

"Then," she said, "here are the contraindications, the reasons for not taking this product. 1. Patients with thrombophlebitis—that's blood clots—or with a history of thrombophlebitis or pulmonary embolism. 2. Liver dysfunction or disease. 3. Patients with known or suspected carcinoma of breast or genital organs." Kathryn read the last with particular emphasis.

"May I see that, Mrs. Huffman?" Baylor rose and went over to her.

"Of course." She handed it to Mike, her attorney, who glanced at it and then gave it to Baylor. He looked the printed leaflet over as he returned to his seat.

"This is an insert from a carton of. . . ."

"Mordrine," she supplied.

"Containing many pill containers?"

"That's right. Medication that's prescribed by a physician has a label that only tells the patient how much to take and how often to take it. Only the medicines you buy without a prescription—over-the-counter medicines—have warnings on the container. The doctors can look up a prescription drug in the *Physicians' Desk Reference Book* or in the literature the drug companies give them. The druggist can learn about it from the one printed insert that comes in each carton of a prescription drug. The customer—the patient—doesn't see anything."

Baylor's questioning continued, "Now, after you saw Dr. Canaris and you began to take the Mordrine, did you go to any other doctor?"

"I saw Dr. Lawrence on September 6, 1968. I saw him because I found a lump in my left breast. Dr. Lawrence took me off the Mordrine."

"You took the Mordrine, at the most, for one month?"

"One menstrual cycle."

"When had you noticed the lump on your breast?"

"Approximately two weeks after I saw Dr. Canaris. I didn't pay much attention to it at first, because I had just seen a gynecologist."

"What breast was it on?"

"The left."

"You felt it yourself?"

"My husband actually called it to my attention. It was something we regarded as being a milk gland."

"Are you quite sure then you had not noticed it before two weeks after you saw Dr. Canaris?" Baylor persisted.

"Yes, I am certain. It was definitely about two weeks later."

"Why are you so certain of that?"

"Because I remember thinking to myself, 'I just saw Dr. Canaris two weeks ago. This lump can't be anything significant.' In other words, I had just seen a gynecologist who had examined my breasts and I felt if there was anything significant there, he would have found it in his examination."

"I'm trying to find out why it is that the two weeks sticks in your mind," Baylor persisted.

"That is why. I remember thinking two weeks is not a very long time."

"How about ten days?"

"Objection," Mike Jefferson said.

"You referred to two weeks," Baylor continued. "What is there about two weeks?"

Kathryn had tested the lawyer's frustration threshold. "You are right," she said. "I should say approximately two weeks."

"Am I correct then, you are giving us your best approximation and you really don't know exactly?" Baylor asked as if he had won a major victory.

"That's correct," replied Kathryn, obviously concerned about why this was so important to Baylor.

He went on, "At the time you were examined by Dr. Canaris, did he not report anything to you of that nature?"

"He told me I was perfectly healthy—as far as my breasts were concerned. He said the problem was in my mind; that I was imagining the pain in my breasts. And that I was imagining my nausea and headaches and acne."

"Had you yourself felt anything in your breast before your husband mentioned it?"

"No."

"You said something about a milk gland. What do you mean by that?"

"We talked about what the lump might be. My husband said it must be an enlarged milk gland due to my period."

"Did you go back to see Dr. Canaris about this?"

"No."

"You then went to see Dr. Lawrence?"

"Yes, I saw him."

"On September 6, 1968?"

"Yes."

"Did you go because of the lump or did you go for something else?"

"For the lump, because it didn't go away. I was beginning to get worried. I wondered if I had breast cancer." Her face became serious as she recalled the incident. "Then I thought—I might lose my breast—and even die. . . ."

"During the time you were taking Mordrine did your symptoms stay the same or did they change in any way?" Baylor asked as he cut her off.

"The symptoms seemed, in fact, to be going away. I had a very bloated feeling that was new, but the headaches and the nausea subsided. I don't know about the acne. It was too soon to tell."

"You said that you saw Dr. Canaris on August 5th, the date you got the prescription filled. Your husband noticed the lump in your breast approximately two weeks later. You did not see Dr. Lawrence until September 6th?"

"Right."

"You continued to take the Mordrine?"

"Yes."

"When you saw Dr. Lawrence, what did you say to him and what did he say to you?"

"I said, 'There's something on my breast' and he examined it. He said, 'There is no doubt in my mind that this is a benign cyst.' He asked me what kind of contraceptive I was using. I said I was taking Mordrine. He said, 'Well, you better get off of that, because it will feed a cyst. I suggest you get off of it for about a month or so. I am going on vacation. Come back in one month and by that time the cyst should dry up and go away.' He said it was not uncommon for young women to have benign cysts in their breasts and the birth control pill could feed them and make them grow. I said, 'Great! I'm glad there's nothing wrong!' I felt so relieved!''

"Did you get off The Pill?"

"Yes, right away. That day I stopped taking it. I never took it again."

"Your total exposure to Mordrine was between August 5, 1968, and September 6, 1968?"

"Yes."

"And your total exposure to the other pill was from the latter part of May or April?"

"The latter part of April."

"Up through August first or so?"

"Yes."

"You took approximately three cycles of Cyclemide and one cycle of Mordrine?"

"Yes."

"The first evidence of any lump appeared about two weeks after you saw Dr. Canaris at which time there was no evidence of any lump?"

"Right."

"Now, when you were taking this Mordrine you said your symptoms changed?"

"The headaches and the nausea seemed to be diminishing."

"How about the acne?"

"No, I still had acne."

"Did that ultimately go away after you stopped taking The Pill?"

"Eventually."

"How about the soreness in your breasts, did that continue after you stopped taking the Mordrine?"

"That let up. It began to stop."

"Am I correct all the symptoms you had began to subside during the time you took Mordrine?"

"Yes."

"Did you tell your husband what Dr. Lawrence had said?"

"Yes, I did."

"What did your husband say?"

"I think he said, 'Oh, yes, I guess that's right.' He agreed with Dr. Lawrence. There was no fight or anything about it. He said he would use a condom for birth control. I think my husband was relieved that there was nothing seriously wrong with me."

Chapter Four

Later, October 24, 1970.

Baylor continued his questioning, bringing out details regarding Kathryn's breast tumor.

"About this lump in your breast, did it change size or shape? Or did it stay the same?"

"It got bigger during the month Dr. Lawrence told me to wait. It continued to grow during the month I got off The Pill."

"Did you go to see Dr. Lawrence again?"

"Yes, October 10, 1968."

"What did you say and what did he say?"

"I said, 'The lump in my breast has gotten bigger.' He said, 'Yes, it has.' " Kathryn paused as if the doctor's words were still haunting her. "Dr. Lawrence said, 'It is just a fibroid tumor and it can be drained or surgically removed, or we can just let it stay around. If you want to have it surgically removed, see Dr. Ivan Frederick.' There was no urgency in his manner. Then he added, 'You can tell your husband and parents that no one is going to cut your breast off.' "

"You said that after Dr. Lawrence told you in September to stop using The Pill, you talked with your husband and he agreed with Dr. Lawrence at that point?"

"Yes."

"Did he, as a prospective doctor, say anything about whether or not Dr. Lawrence should take a biopsy of the tissue in the lump? A microscopic examination?"

"No, he did not."

"After you saw Dr. Lawrence in October, did you discuss with your husband what Dr. Lawrence had told you?"

"I told him what Dr. Lawrence told me."

"Did your husband say anything?"

"No, he did not have any opinion, really. His own opinion was if I did go to see a surgeon, I should go to one at Barnard, the hospital where he was. He could get professional courtesy. He was concerned about the money. I told him I was sure my parents would pay for it if necessary."

"What did you say to your parents?"

"I was worried that if I had the tumor removed, it would leave a scar, and that would disfigure my breast. I wanted a good surgeon. My parents felt I should get several medical opinions. Then I went to Dr. Frederick."

"When did you go to see Dr. Frederick?"

"October, 1968. I don't have the exact date."

"Sometime after October 10th?"

"Yes. I also went to see Dr. Halsey. . . ."

"You're a little too fast for me. What did Dr. Frederick say?"

"He thought I ought to have the tumor removed."

"Did he give you any opinion as to what kind of tumor he thought it was?"

"He said it seemed to be the kind that in most cases is benign."

"But he left open the area of a possibility that it was a cancerous tumor?"

"Yes. If you want the exact reason why I didn't want to have Dr. Frederick as my surgeon, I can tell you. I was ready to, but when it came to signing the authorization for surgery, his name wasn't on it. I said to the nurse, 'Would you please put Dr. Frederick's name on this authorization? Then I'll be glad to sign it.' She said, 'We don't bother with that.' I said, 'I am not going to bother with you.' I walked out. There was no provision that he would be the doctor who did the surgery. It could have been an intern or a resident at the hospital who would cut me. I didn't know. There was nothing for me to go on legally."

Baylor peered at her sharply and, looking down at her, said, "You're not a lawyer, are you?"

Kathryn turned his put-down around. "I'm getting a doctorate in international law."

He appeared shocked by her answer. "You are getting a doctorate in international law?" he asked.

"That's my major field," she replied.

"Have you taken any courses at all?" he asked.

"I have completed *all* my courses for the doctorate," Kathryn answered.

"Where are you getting your doctorate?" Baylor asked. "At what school?"

"At Harvard University. That's where I got my Master's in Public Law and Government."

"What do you have to do now before you get your doctorate?" Baylor persisted.

"I've completed all my courses; I've passed my written examination. I've passed my language examinations in French and Latin. Now I'm developing my master's thesis into a doctoral dissertation. And I have to take the oral examination," Kathryn explained.

Baylor decided it was wise to drop this line of questioning. He returned to his notes. Raising his head, after a moment, he continued, "Did you ask Dr. Frederick why he did not put his name on the surgery authorization form?"

"He was too busy to talk with me. The nurse said he never did it."

"You were not in the hospital. You were just in his office?"

"Yes."

"Did he examine you?"

"He looked at my breast."

Annoyance took over again as he said, "I am not asking you if he looked at your breast. I am asking you if he examined you other than your breast."

"No, just the breast."

"When he examined the breast, can you tell me, if you know, approximately what size the tumor was at that time?"

"I'm really not competent to give a judgment on that."

"You of course, had been feeling yourself."

"It had grown. I don't know what size."

"It was larger than it had been when you first noticed it?"

"Yes."

"Did he recommend you have it taken out immediately?"

"No, he said there was no urgency."

"How long were you there?"

"I waited for two hours beyond my appointment time to see him. I saw him for about fifteen minutes and I was rushed out to sign an authorization."

"What do you mean by rushed out?"

"Well, he said, 'How do you do?' He took a look at the tumor. He said, 'Very good. I think it is probably benign. I will take it out if you want me to. Go see my nurse.'"

"Didn't he tell you of any dangers that might go with taking it out?"

"No, he did not."

"Didn't he tell you anything about the danger of a frozen section before he took it out?"

"No. Nobody told me about any danger involved in removing the tumor. In fact, this is the first time I've ever heard of a 'danger of a frozen section.' A frozen section is simply an examination of tissue that has been removed and then frozen."

Baylor was annoyed that he had lost control of the situation. "I am asking you, did he tell you that?"

"No, he didn't."

"Where did you go after you left there?"

"I went to see Dr. Halsey at Barnard Hospital."

"Before we get to him, were you then living in Englewood Cliffs, New Jersey?"

"In October, yes."

"Did your husband come home every night?"

"He was in the hospital every third night and every other weekend, I believe."

"Did you discuss with him or your parents or anybody the results of your visit to Dr. Frederick?"

"Yes. They were all disgusted with the way Dr. Frederick treated me. My husband was anxious, of course, for me to use somebody at Barnard Hospital."

"When you discussed it with your husband, did he say anything other than that he would like you to see somebody at Barnard Hospital?"

"No, he didn't have time to get involved with my condition."

Baylor turned to Mike Jefferson and in an aggrieved tone, eyeglasses in hand, said, "You know, Mr. Jefferson, I don't mean to be presumptuous, but a lot of these answers have material added on which I do not think is responsive. I would like to make a note in the record so we will have no difficulty in the future. There may be times when we may have to object to the non-responsiveness and ask that they be stricken in some instances. I would like to reserve that right without being presumptuous."

"It's all right. I think your objection is well noted, Mr. Baylor," Mike replied. "I would urge you, Mrs. Huffman, to try to answer the question, and if there's something else you think may be interesting, don't mention it if it really isn't a direct response to the question."

"All right, I'll try," Kathryn replied.

Mike continued, "Counsel does want a full and complete answer to the question, but he does not want any question to be a take-off for a speech. Give him a complete answer, then stop."

Baylor again took up his questioning, "Mrs. Huffman, were there difficulties between you and your husband from the time you were married right up until the time you had this operation?"

"No, nothing significant."

"Mrs. Huffman," Baylor continued. "You have told us something about your husband. You described him as a rather dominating individual."

"Yes."

"Even before you had the radical mastectomy, were you and he having arguments with each other?"

"Yes, we had some arguments."

"I won't pursue that any further at this moment. Mrs. Huffman, the next doctor you went to see after Dr. Frederick was whom?"

"Dr. Halsey."

"Where is he located?"

"Barnard Hospital."

"Who recommended him?"

"My husband."

"Incidentally, may I go back again, excuse me, to Dr. Frederick. Did he tell you what, in his opinion, was the cause of the lump in your breast?"

"No."

"Did you ask him?"

"No."

"Did you tell him that you'd been taking these birth control pills?"

"I don't remember."

"How soon after you saw Dr. Frederick did you see Dr. Halsey? Do you recall that visit?"

"I recall that visit. I don't remember the date, but it was in October, 1968, soon after I saw Dr. Frederick."

"Did you discuss with your husband the results of your visit to Dr. Halsey?"

"Yes."

"What did he say?"

"Well, Conrad was pleased that I thought Dr. Halsey was a nice man. He really didn't have an opinion of his own about whether I should have an operation or not. He thought that if I wanted to have it done, Dr. Halsey should do it."

"Did you see any other doctor thereafter?"

"Yes, I saw Dr. Julius Wilkinson on November 2, 1968, at the Lyle Medical Group and I was impressed by him, much more than I had been impressed by the other surgeons. He said he was very sure the tumor was a benign cyst, but recommended that it be removed. I remember telling him I had been on birth control pills and he said birth control pills are known to contribute to the growth of breast tumors. I was impressed by him, and then and there decided to have it done. I was told to go downstairs to the office and make the necessary arrangements. There was no rush put on it by Dr. Wilkinson. I was not an emergency patient. I wasn't to be operated on until sixteen days later, so obviously it was no real rush, if I had to wait sixteen days."

"During this time, you were not taking either of these pills?"

"That's correct."

"During the sixteen days, did your lump get larger?"

"Not that I recall."

"Did you discuss with your husband that you were going to be operated on?"

"Yes."

"Did he know Dr. Wilkinson?"

"No, he didn't know him."

"What hospital were you going to have it done at?"

"Dillard Hospital."

"Was it ultimately done there?"

"Yes."

"Up to this time, having had this lump in your breast and having this apprehension about taking birth control pills, hadn't you done any reading on the subject at all?" Baylor asked.

"I don't think I did any reading between the time that Dr. Lawrence saw the tumor and the time I had the radical mastectomy because I was involved with preparing for my examination at the university, trying to get my apartment furnished, and making appointments to see surgeons. I was too busy and too concerned about my health and my university work to go into medical research."

"Everybody had told you it was most probably benign."

"Yes, but I was still concerned. I was worried about the scar that was going to be left after the surgery."

"What was the reason that you were so concerned about the scar?"

"It is possible I could have thought I might be less attractive to my husband after surgery since he thought women's breasts were important. My breasts were important to me also."

"Now, you did not read anything on this subject until after you had the radical mastectomy? Is that correct?" Baylor appeared to have some anxiety regarding this subject.

"Nothing of any significance. I might have seen something in the paper."

"I want to know what you read, if anything. Whether you think it was significant may or may not be the test."

"No, I don't believe I had time."

"What were you doing?"

"I was studying at the law library. I was running around seeing surgeons. I was running the household, you know, shopping, cleaning and cooking. And I was worrying."

"You only saw three surgeons: Dr. Frederick, Dr. Halsey and Dr. Wilkinson?"

"Yes. This was all within two months. To me it seemed like I was running around. You certainly must know, Mr. Baylor, that it usually takes several weeks to get to see a surgeon for an examination. I saw three surgeons within twenty working days. There's a waiting period from the time you call for an appointment until the surgeon sees you."

"You were obviously a very studious young lady, and you didn't get curious in view of your worry to read something about this subject?" Baylor asked, ignoring Kathryn's comment.

She answered, "I had read about The Pill before that in just one article that appeared in *The New York Times*. Dr. Lawrence had told me The Pill could cause the tumor to grow, and he also said if I stopped taking The Pill, the tumor should go away. I felt quite certain that there was a relationship between The Pill and the tumor. I figured as soon as I got out of the hospital, I was going to do some reading on the subject. I wanted to get the surgery over with first."

"You wanted to get it over with, but you went to three different doctors."

"Well, I wanted to get it over with but I didn't want to jeopardize my health while I was doing it."

"By the way, by the time you got to Dr. Wilkinson did you still have headaches, nausea, acne and soreness of your breasts, or had that all disappeared?" Baylor asked.

"I think the soreness of the breasts had disappeared. The acne, I think, remained."

"Mrs. Huffman, when you went to Dillard Hospital, did you give a history at the time you went in?"

Pain and exhaustion were beginning to show in Kathryn's face. She sipped water, bracing herself for the recital of her history. "Yes."

"Do you remember what you told them?"

"I gave them my medical history."

Annoyed, Baylor said, "I know that! I am asking you, do you remember what you told them?"

Kathryn wouldn't rise to his annoyance. She spoke quietly, "I told them everything that they wanted to know. The resident doctor came in and asked me questions about my childhood diseases, what operations I'd had, all of that."

"Did you tell him you had been taking birth control pills?"

"Yes, I did. I also told the nurses. One of the nurses told me there had been an alarming increase in the number of young women coming into the hospital with tumors in their breasts, who had taken the birth control pills."

"Do you remember the name of the nurse who told you that?"

"Yes, her name is Inga Robbins. I'll never forget her and the support she gave me at that time."

"I must comment and make a motion on that, the last answer," he said, making a note. "Did you tell the resident who took your history that you were taking birth control pills?"

"Yes. I was telling everybody."

"How long were you in the hospital before the operation was done? Do you recall that?"

"Two days."

"You went to the hospital on what date?"

"I went in on a Sunday. It was done on a Monday. The operation was performed on November 18, 1968. There were two operations, one to remove the tumor and then two days later, after they concluded the tumor was malignant, they performed the radical mastectomy."

"Mr. Jefferson, will you get the exact date," demanded Baylor.

"The diary indicates November 18, 1968, was a Monday," Jefferson said as he glanced at the page in his client's diary.

"That was the first one," Kathryn said.

"And the 20th was a Wednesday," Jefferson added.

Baylor motioned to Kathryn to continue. "The 18th and the 20th were the days of my operations. I went in on Sunday, the 17th."

"When did you learn that the tumor was not benign?"

"I think it was Tuesday morning."

"That would be the 19th of November, 1968. Is that correct?"

"Yes."

"Who told you that?"

"Dr. Aaron."

"Who?"

"Dr. Aaron."

"He wasn't the doctor who operated, was he?"

"No, he was not. He told me because he felt that I knew him

better than Dr. Wilkinson at that time. Dr. Aaron had recommended Dr. Wilkinson to me."

"What did he say? I know this may be painful to you, but I must know, please. What did he say?"

"Well, first of all, I had a feeling when he called that it was malignant, otherwise he wouldn't have called."

"He called you on the telephone?" Baylor asked, appearing rather surprised.

"Yes. He told me that I was intelligent. When somebody tells you that you are intelligent, you know you are going to hear bad news. He said they had about five pathologists from Memorial Hospital and Dillard Hospital doing frozen sections on my tumor and it was malignant beyond any shadow of doubt."

"He told you this on the phone?" Baylor again asked in disbelief.

"Yes."

"Were you alone when this happened?"

"I was with my nurse, Mrs. Robbins."

"Then what did he say to you?"

"He told me that Dr. Wilkinson was the best surgeon he could think of to perform the operation, and that it was up to me to decide what would happen, but there was only one decision to be made, and that was to have the radical mastectomy—to have the breast and all the connected muscle and lymph glands removed. That was the whole thing." Kathryn looked down at her left arm and hand, swollen and bandaged.

"This news, I am sure, upset you."

A tear crept down her cheek. She quickly erased it with her finger. She spoke softly, "Of course." She was silent a moment, and then took a deep breath. "My family, I think, was told before I knew. When they came in, I didn't have to tell them."

"What about your husband, what did he have to say?"

Her hand trembled a little as she lifted the glass to drink some water. "I don't remember seeing my husband too often in the hospital. He came in about every other day. I don't recall his being there that day. I honestly don't remember what he said. Is that a good answer?''

Baylor ignored her question. ''Can you tell us what your mother and father said to you?''

''I don't think anybody said anything really. They came in with Dr. Wilkinson. Dr. Wilkinson explained why the operation had to be performed. It was all kind of scientific.''

''Did you ever ask Dr. Wilkinson at any time subsequent to the operation about what had caused the malignancy?''

''Yes, I did. He told me the birth control pill could definitely trigger a tumor and cause its growth. He said The Pill could cause a tumor to grow where it might have lain dormant indefinitely or for a number of years. He also said it was possible to transform a benign tumor into a malignancy by a hormone reaction.''

''So that what he was telling you then, as I understand what you have told me, and you correct me if I am wrong . . . Dr. Wilkinson said that taking the birth control pills could cause a tumor to grow as well as to change a benign tumor into cancer?''

''Yes, he said that was an example of the harm that medical technology can cause. It was his opinion that my illness was due to a harmful reaction to the estrogen contained in the birth control pill. When I attended one of the Senate meetings, I heard Dr. Cutler say that estrogen in The Pill can stimulate the growth of breast cancer.''

Baylor glanced over at the papers Kathryn was reviewing. ''Do you have anything in writing to that effect?'' he asked.

''I have a copy of the speech Dr. Cutler delivered to the Senate Subcommittee on Monopoly hearings. Dr. Cutler said: 'In clinical practice, we avoid the use of estrogens for fear of increasing the activity of existing disease or stimulating the growth of clinically latent foci of breast cancer.' ''

''Then this radical mastectomy was done on your left side?'' Baylor asked.

''Yes,'' Kathryn replied.

"Do you know how long you were hospitalized for that?"

"About ten days."

"After that where did you go?"

"I went to my parents' home."

"Why didn't you return to your apartment?"

"My husband said he didn't have the time to give me the attention I might need."

"Did your husband remain at your apartment?"

"Yes."

"How long did you stay at the home of your mother and father?"

"Until the present day."

"Off the record," Baylor announced. The hour was late and Kathryn was visibly exhausted. The taking of the deposition was adjourned until Friday, October 30, 1970, at 9:30 in the morning.

Chapter Five

October 26, 1970.

Huffman, Kathryn
Physicians' Hospital #524 06

Kathryn Huffman was seen in consultation by Dr. Joshua Alexander of the Neurology Department. A nerve block was attempted to block the intense pain caused by an advanced malignancy. The attempt was unsuccessful and the patient was discharged the same day.

October 28, 1970.

Huffman, Kathryn Stuart
Memorial Hospital #102216

The patient was seen by Dr. Philip Hakon. Arrangements were made for a surgical incision to be performed in the area of the affected lymph nodes to determine whether radiation is the treatment of choice.

October 30, 1970.

The second session of Kathryn's deposition, scheduled for October 30 in Michael Jefferson's office, was postponed to Tuesday, November 3, at 9:40 A.M., at the request of Mr. Baylor and Mr. Griffith.

November 3, 1970.

A nip of fall was in the air, and the sky was more overcast than usual.

Kathryn was seated again at the table facing the defense lawyers in Mike's office. She was like a beautiful ray of sunlight against the drab gray outside and the somber attire of the lawyers. She wore her powder-blue pants suit; a reminder of happier days. She tried to appear composed, but anyone could see she was in great pain and could hardly sit upright. It was determination alone that enabled her to make her appearance today.

Mike had been alerted that Kathryn could not walk without falling this morning, but he insisted that she appear, even if it was necessary to call an ambulance. Time was running out. . . .

The court reporter opened the second session on Kathryn's deposition:

"Kathryn Stuart Huffman, the plaintiff, having been duly sworn, testifies," he paused as he read from the notes: "Direct examination by Baylor continuing."

"Mrs. Huffman, I would . . ."

"Mr. Baylor, may I interrupt you for just a moment," Mike Jefferson said, "to note on the record that we have a little extra problem in terms of the effect of some medication."

"Do you want this on the record?" Baylor asked.

"Yes," Jefferson replied. "We can anticipate that it may take Mrs. Huffman a little extra time to answer. I think Mrs. Huffman is competent to proceed with the deposition, but she had some medication last night and still feels its effects this morning. It might make her somewhat slower in responding, as compared to the last session."

"I think we ought to clarify on the record," Baylor stated, "that if there is any question at all of the lady's competence to answer any question, to completely understand the question and respond, then I am concluding the deposition right here and now. We do not want to be faced with an eventual situation where the plaintiff can claim that she wasn't mentally or physically competent to answer any question. That should be settled now. I recognize the lady may not feel well. If she doesn't, of course, we will cease immediately.''

"Mr. Baylor, I am satisfied from preliminary questioning of the plaintiff this morning that she is competent. If I didn't think so, I would not propose, as I do, that we proceed. I am merely suggesting that defense counsel understand that perhaps we will require a few more seconds, and that perhaps the questions could be put a little more slowly. If at any time I feel, or the plaintiff feels, she is not competent to proceed, we will certainly say so and I think we will have to stop the depositions. I do not anticipate that is going to happen.''

Baylor said, "Off the record."

Kathryn and her mother were asked to leave the room.

A few minutes later, they were told to return and Baylor continued, "I think the record should reveal we have had a conference with Mr. Jefferson and counsel outside of the presence of Mrs. Huffman and her mother. Mr. Jefferson also had a conference with Mrs. Huffman and her mother and has been advised that the plaintiff has taken some medication last night because intense pain was keeping her from sleeping, and that she feels, apparently based upon her experience, that within a half an hour or so, whatever drowsiness or lethargy that she may have at the moment will be cleared up. We have all agreed, with the consent of Mr. Jefferson, to wait an hour, at which time we will check with the young lady and see how she feels and make a determination at that time as to whether to proceed with these depositions. Is that statement agreeable to you?''

"Yes, that's agreeable to the plaintiff. Thank you, gentlemen, I appreciate your cooperation,'' Mike replied.

One hour later.

"Shall we start?" Baylor inquired.

"By all means," Mike responded.

"Mrs. Huffman, it is now five minutes to eleven, and as you know, we adjourned for some period of time to give you an opportunity to see whether or not you felt clearer, and so forth. Do you feel better now?"

Kathryn may not have felt better, but she was more alert. "I'm ready," she replied.

Baylor continued, "Do you have any difficulty in understanding what I have just said?"

"No," she answered.

"Did you have any difficulty in answering the question that I just asked you?"

"No." Her answer was a little louder.

"Do we understand you took some medication last night which made you perhaps drowsy or sleepy this morning?"

"Yes."

"And did you take an unusual amount of it?"

"No. I took what I take every night. It was the same medication."

"Does it have the same effect upon you daily?"

"Usually I sleep until around noon, so I sleep it off."

"In other words, you are just up earlier this morning than you normally are. Is that correct?"

"Yes."

"Would you feel any better if we waited until noon?"

"If I had been sleeping all this time, I would have slept it off, but it's too late for that now."

"If you feel at any time that you want to stop because you either are tired or you feel sleepy or anything of that nature, will you advise us of that?"

"Yes."

"Now, in the hour that we have been gone, from the time we

started until now, have you been walking around, talking or what? What have you been doing?''

Kathryn seemed amazed by his question. "I don't think that's relevant.''

"Whether you think it is relevant or not, I am asking the question," Baylor growled.

"Kathryn," Mike Jefferson said, as he leaned over and touched her hand, "tell everything you have been doing for the last hour.''

"We've been sitting around. I've been walking around." She paused, then continued, "I went to the ladies' room and urinated." She paused again. "I wiped myself, I washed my hands. . . ."

"I didn't want all those details," Baylor interrupted, his face flushing.

She continued, "You demanded an answer and I am giving it to you. I had a Vicks Medicated Cough Drop and drank some water. Mr. Jefferson and I talked about history and current events.''

"Did you understand the conversation when you talked about history?''

"Yes.''

"Do you feel now that you are more aware at the present time than you were an hour ago?''

"Yes.''

"Mrs. Huffman," he began, after glancing at his notes, "I think when we left you last time you had gone to your parents' home. Is that correct?''

"Yes.''

"How long did you remain at home with your parents after this radical mastectomy? We don't have to have the precise date.''

"Until the present time.''

"What time are we talking about? When the radical mastectomy took place? When was that?''

"That was November 20th.''

"Of 1968?''

"1968, yes.''

"I think you told us the other day that sometime in January of 1969 you told your husband you were ready to go back and live together, but you could not live together as man and wife and engage in sexual activities because you still had some residual bleeding."

"*He* said we couldn't live together. I told him that I couldn't have sexual relations with him, and he said then we couldn't live together."

"You had made the offer to go back?"

"Yes, I did."

"And because of the circumstances, and your feelings about sex, he said you couldn't go back together?"

"He wouldn't allow me to!"

"How long did he remain in that apartment? Do you know that?"

"As far as I know, until May, 1969."

"Where did he go in May of 1969? Do you know?"

"I have no idea."

"When did you last see your husband face to face?"

"That day in March of 1969 I told you about," she reminded Baylor.

"I think you told us the other day, it was January, 1969."

"January, 1969, is when I said I would come back to the apartment. I last saw him on March 17, 1969."

Baylor flipped backwards through his notes and then looked up at Kathryn. "Did you talk to your mother and father or either of them about this meeting with your husband at which he gave you the ultimatum?"

"I talked to both of them."

"At the same time?"

"I don't recall. I know my father told me that my husband spoke to him on two occasions that evening. The first time was before my husband went into my room and the second time was after he came out. I don't remember if I talked to both of my parents at the same time."

"What did your father say that your husband said he was going to say to you?"

The question sounded like a riddle, one that Baylor wanted her to figure out for herself.

"Excuse me?" Kathryn asked.

Baylor rephrased the question in his monotonous voice, "What did your father tell you that your husband told him that he was going to say to you?"

"Conrad told him he was going to give me an ultimatum—that I had to have intercourse with him or he'd have our marriage annulled. My father said, 'Well, that's like abandoning a sinking ship.' My husband said to my father, 'Even a drowning rat deserves a chance to get off a sinking ship.' My father replied, 'Well, if the shoe fits. . . .' "

Baylor cut her off. "Have you had any communication with your husband at all except through the service of these divorce papers?" he said, waving them at her from across the table.

"No."

"So you have neither talked with your husband personally, nor talked with him by phone, nor had any correspondence with him since the service of these papers. Is that correct?"

"Correct."

Baylor consulted his notes before continuing. "I gather at the time we are talking about now, you were in your parents' house and going back and forth to visit the doctor on a number of occasions that you've told us about?"

"Yes."

"Are we talking about March, April, or February of 1969? Can you help us a little bit on that?"

"Through March of 1969," she explained. "In the beginning of March, I had an attack of gastroenteritis. I was in bed for a week."

"Who treated you for the gastroenteritis?"

"Dr. Julius Wilkinson. That was March 6, 1969."

"How did you determine the date as March 6, 1969?"

"From Dr. Wilkinson's bill."

"Now, going back, please, during the time that you were in bed with this gastroenteritis, how was this pain in your chest?"

"It was worse. It was worse, because all the vomiting I did made the bleeding more profuse and that gave me more pain."

Baylor looked over at Kathryn, then went on, "Now, Mrs. Huffman, you have given us your opinion, in spite of the fact you are not a doctor, about what caused the bleeding. Did you ask Dr. Wilkinson after you got over the gastroenteritis what caused the increase in bleeding?"

"I don't remember doing so," she replied.

"By this time you knew you had a malignancy."

"Of course, yes."

"Did you at any time up to this point, when you had gastroenteritis, ask Dr. Wilkinson whether or not in his opinion this pain was related to or caused by cancer?"

"I believe that I did ask him if it was possible that I still had cancer, because I still had so much pain."

"What was his answer?"

"He said the tests for cancer were all negative."

"Now, Mrs. Huffman, as I understand from what you said the other day, you and Conrad Huffman discussed the use of contraceptives prior to your marriage? Is that correct?"

"Yes, Conrad and I began talking about using contraceptives. He wanted me to take The Pill. I said I'd discuss this further with my family physician."

Baylor, going back to his notes, asked, "Did you ever ask Dr. Lawrence whether or not there was any danger of getting cancer from these birth control pills?"

Kathryn stopped to think carefully about this question. "I reminded Dr. Lawrence that I previously had a benign tumor of the parotid gland. That's the salivary gland, near your ear. I was concerned that that might be a reason for not taking The Pill."

"Did you ever ask Dr. Lawrence whether or not there was any fear that you would get cancer from taking The Pill?" Baylor repeated.

"Not cancer, no."

"You told us the other day that the doctor had not recommended The Pill for your mother."

"That's right."

"Did you discuss with your mother why he had not recommended The Pill?"

"Yes."

"Why?"

"Dr. Lawrence felt she might have a fibroid tumor."

"Your mother might have had a fibroid tumor?"

"Yes, of the uterus. He just felt it wasn't a good idea for her to use it."

After consulting his notes again, Baylor asked, "Did there come a time when the wound finally healed up?"

"Eventually."

"When was that?"

"I would say approximately in April of 1970—one and a half years after the surgery!"

"Did you go once a week to see Dr. Wilkinson all during this period of time?"

"No. I stopped seeing Dr. Wilkinson in March of 1969."

"Why?"

"He had suggested before that I could go back into the hospital and have another operation to make the wound heal. He would make a new incision, taking enough skin this time so the wound could heal. I was willing to undergo surgery again—anything so I could heal properly! But then in March—March, 1969—he decided instead that I should just apply salt water soaks to my wound and wait for that to heal it. I felt he couldn't really do anything more for me, and that I should see another doctor about the bleeding."

"Did you consult another doctor about your condition?"

"Yes."

"What doctor did you see after Dr. Wilkinson?"

"Dr. Daniel Ashoka, at University Hospital."

"Did you tell him that you had had a radical mastectomy?"

"I didn't have to! He could see my breast had been removed."

Baylor cleared his throat noisily. "How many times did you see him?"

"Eight times."

"Over what period of time?"

"From March, 1969, to November, 1969."

"Would you tell us what you said to him when you first saw him?"

"I said, 'Please try to heal my wound.' "

"Did you tell him about the solution Dr. Wilkinson told you to use?"

"Yes. He did not think the saline solution was proper treatment for my problem."

"Did he examine you?"

"Yes. He examined me and he tried to cauterize the wound. He felt that by burning the raw tissues, they would heal. This is a procedure used in India. Dr. Ashoka is Indian."

"Was that painful, that cauterizing?"

"Not any more painful than when Dr. Wilkinson tore away original scar tissue each time I saw him."

"Did Dr. Ashoka repeat the cauterization on each visit?"

"Yes."

"How long did the treatments take?"

"Just a minute."

"Did it cure the condition?"

"No, it did not."

"When Dr. Ashoka would do this cauterization or burning treatment did he wrap your breast up in any way after it was over?"

"You mean my breast area. My breast had been cut off. After Dr. Ashoka cauterized the wound he put a four-by-four gauze pad over the opening in my chest."

"How often was that changed?"

"He asked me to change that every day, and I did."

''Did you put any medication on it at all?''

''No.''

''Did it finally cure or did it not cure?''

''No, it did not. Finally I went to see another doctor.''

''Did you still have this pain that you had earlier which you told us about that was deep inside?''

''No. By this time I just had numbness.''

''Can you tell us when it was that the pain had left you, approximately? I don't expect you to know the exact date.''

''It's very difficult to say. I think the major pain left in January, 1969. That is why I thought I could go back to my husband. However, I still could not stand to be touched. That area was still terribly sensitive to touch.''

''What doctor did you see after Dr. Ashoka?''

''Dr. Mark Allen.''

''What is Dr. Allen's specialty? Do you know that?''

''He specializes in breast cancer.''

''Did you have a discussion with him?''

''Yes, we talked about everything that had happened.''

''Did he ask you who had performed the radical mastectomy?''

''Yes. After two visits he said he could not help me. He referred me to Dr. Peter Gates, who is a dermatologist. It was through Dr. Gates' efforts that I eventually healed. I have a copy of his letter for the court record,'' she said, as Mike handed the letter to Baylor.

From the Record
December 4, 1969

Dear Dr. Allen:

Thank you for referring Mrs. Kathryn Stuart Huffman. I took an antibiotic sensitivity test from the wound and for the time being applied a special cream solution in the hope that the low grade infection is caused by gram-negative bacillus, which will respond to this cream.

Mrs. Huffman's husband's behavior, in my opinion, has been insensitive and inhumane toward her. I am, by means of this letter, going on record that I will be willing to testify as an expert witness on her behalf at the forthcoming divorce trial. Her physical condition during this past year contraindicated sexual involvement as demanded by her husband.

Sincerely yours,
Peter Gates, M.D.

"Did you see any other doctor after you saw Dr. Gates?"

"Yes."

"Who was that?"

"I began to see Dr. Alvin Engle on April 22, 1970, when my arm started to swell."

"Which arm?"

Kathryn lifted her arm at the elbow so that he could get a better look at the elastic wrapping. It was quite obvious to everyone there that she could not move her left arm without a great deal of pain. Her face grew pale and beaded with perspiration. "My left arm became quite swollen," she said, "and I had a stabbing pain in the left shoulder. I discussed this with Dr. Allen when I saw him in February. He said radical mastectomy patients often get swelling and have these complaints. He told me not to worry about it. But it kept getting worse—it got to be so painful that my mother insisted I see a neurologist. She felt a neurologist might know something about the pain and how to help me. I needed help! Mother knew of Dr. Engle by reputation. She heard he was a fine neurologist, and that is why I went to see him."

"When you went to see Dr. Engle, did you give him a full history regarding your condition?"

"Of course."

"You understand that we are going to ask you about your conversation with Dr. Engle as it regarded your experience with Dr. Lawrence or anybody else who had to do with your condition. Is that clear?"

"Yes."

"We are talking about the first time you saw Dr. Engle. According to the piece of paper we have here, that was on April 22, 1970," Baylor said, waving a sheet of paper.

"I want my objection noted to any of these conversations." An attorney named Arnold, who represented Dr. Lawrence, interrupted.

Baylor ignored him. "What did you say to Dr. Engle and what did he say to you?" he asked Kathryn.

"Do you mean the entire hour or two that I spent with him?"

"Whatever time you were there and whatever you can remember."

"I told him I was there because I was in a great deal of pain; he was a neurologist and dealt with pain. I told him honestly that by now I hated physicians—that by this time, I had really *had* it with doctors! I was very hostile in the way I spoke to him. When I told him how I felt toward doctors, he took off his white jacket and said, 'You know something? I hate doctors, too!' He took out a pipe and started to smoke it. He said, 'What can I do for you?' I said, 'Well I wish you could help me with this pain.' He said, 'Who is your doctor?' I said, 'Dr. Read is at the present time.' "

"*Who*?" Dr. Read's name was new to Baylor.

Kathryn spelled it out to him. "Dr. Benjamin Read. He has been my internist since September 13, 1969."

"Okay," said Baylor, noting the name. "Please continue with your discussion with Dr. Engle."

"I told Dr. Engle that I was separated from my husband and was in the process of getting a divorce. I told him about the ultimatum and events leading up to the divorce.

"I told him I felt there was a relationship between The Pill and breast cancer. I told him about my concern for other women on The Pill and how I had tried to alert the American Cancer Society, the American Medical Association, the Food and Drug Administration, a number of Congressmen, and leading specialists to this danger. I told him about one of the Senate Subcommittee meetings

I attended in Washington, D.C., on March 3, 1970, the one at which Dr. Max Cutler reported his findings regarding the relation of the birth control pill to breast cancer.''

"What else did you discuss with Dr. Engle?" Baylor asked.

"I told him that I had made very little progress. Some people were sympathetic, but they were not willing to stand up and be counted. I told him as a last resort I started this suit against the drug firms. I told him the lawyers insisted that I also had to include litigation against the doctors, because the drug firms, in an effort to whitewash themselves, would blame the doctors for being negligent. I told him I expected the doctors to deny negligence, and blame the drug firms for glossing over the possible dangers of The Pill and not making enough information on those dangers available to the public.''

"May I interrupt you here, Mrs. Huffman? Up to now, had Dr. Engle examined you?''

"No, he hadn't. He examined me the next time I saw him.''

"You told him you had taken birth control pills and you felt there was a relationship between your illness and The Pill?''

"Yes, we talked about that.''

"Did he answer that?''

"He said he had been reading that studies were being published concerning mental illness and the birth control pill, and that there might be neurological impairments—nervous system damage—caused by The Pill. He is not a research specialist in this area and did not claim to be. He wanted to know everything there was to know about my trouble with the birth control pills. I gave him a good idea of everything that had happened.

"Dr. Engle said there was nothing emotionally wrong with me. He said he felt that it was all a physical problem and that he wouldn't stop until he got to the bottom of it!''

"What did he say when you told him about your husband's ultimatum that he would divorce you if you didn't have intercourse with him following the radical mastectomy?''

"He said, 'Shit!' ''

"He said what?'' Baylor's glasses literally jumped at the end of his nose.

"He said, 'Shit!' '' Then, seeing the look of disbelief on Baylor's face, she added, ''You do know the word, don't you?

"Dr. Engle was very upset about everything I told him,'' Kathryn went on. ''He thought I had had a rough deal all the way. That it was unethical for Dr. Canaris to tell me that I was neurotic and imagining my symptoms. He felt Dr. Canaris was not competent to make a diagnosis that I was neurotic. He also thought Dr. Canaris was unethical for telling me that I was imagining the side effects from The Pill when the literature in the *Physician's Desk Reference Book* clearly specified the side effects I was having.''

"Did Dr. Engle tell you that in his opinion there was a relationship between taking The Pill and the lump that you got in your breast?''

"No.''

"You only discussed Dr. Lawrence and Dr. Canaris, or did you discuss all the other doctors with him?''

"I gave him a very brief review of all the doctors I had seen.''

"Including Dr. Wilkinson?''

"Yes.''

"On the first occasion you told him about the pain that you had? Did he do anything at all about examining your shoulder?''

"No, he said he would consult with a colleague of his, who was a surgeon, about that.''

"Who is the colleague? Do you know that?''

"Yes. I saw him. He ultimately performed further surgery on me.''

"What is his name?''

"Dr. Robert Buchanan.''

"Did Dr. Engle examine the swelling in your arm?''

"He looked at it, but he did not examine it.''

"Where was the swelling at that time?''

"All through my left arm.''

"When did the swelling first appear?"

"In January of 1970."

"Didn't you ask any doctor what was causing the swelling?"

"I saw Dr. Allen in February of 1970 and discussed the swelling with him. Dr. Allen said radical mastectomy patients usually get swelling in their arms. It's not uncommon."

"Was January the first time you had noticed the swelling?"

"Yes, that's correct."

"The radical mastectomy had been in 1968?"

"Yes, but he said it can occur any time."

"Now, who is Dr. Read?"

"He is my present doctor, an internist," said Kathryn.

"When did you start seeing him about your condition?"

"I started to see Dr. Read in 1969, sometime after my incision ripped open."

"Did you ever ask Dr. Read the cause of your breast cancer?"

"The cause?"

"Yes."

"No, I didn't."

"Did you ever ask him the cause of the swelling in your arm?"

"No. I went to the breast cancer specialist, Dr. Allen, regarding the swelling. Dr. Allen sent his report to Dr. Read. Dr. Allen said it was normal for swelling to occur after a radical mastectomy."

"When you went to see Dr. Read the first time in 1969, what were your complaints at that time?"

"I just went for a routine examination. The surgeons I saw didn't give me routine physical examinations, so I thought I'd better see an internist. I didn't want to use Dr. Lawrence anymore. He'd been rather crude in his speech, like when he said 'Tell your husband and parents no one is going to cut your breast off.' That kind of thing. After my radical mastectomy I knew he was wrong, and decided that Dr. Lawrence really was not a good doctor. Not after he misrepresented The Pill. . . ."

"Did you ever ask Dr. Read if he had any opinion that the birth control pills caused the lump to appear in your breast?"

"I don't remember having done so."

"Did he ever volunteer any opinion as to a causal connection, one way or the other?"

"No."

"You continued, I gather, to see this Dr. Engle on a rather frequent basis?"

"Yes."

"Did Dr. Engle at any time ever examine your arm physically?"

"Yes."

"When did he first do that?"

"I don't know. I believe during the second appointment."

"What did he do when he examined your arm? Tell us what he did."

"He pricked it with a pin. He ran the pin up and down the arm and he made certain pin pricks in my hand to determine whether the nerve sensations were dull or sharp. He concluded that—"

"Excuse me," Baylor interrupted. "I'm asking only for what he did, not what he concluded." He mopped his face with a handkerchief. "Now, is that all Dr. Engle did?" Baylor inquired, "just run the pin up and down your arm? Did he give you any other test to your arm: raise it, lower it, put it back of you, turn your hand in one direction or the other?"

"No. I don't think so."

Again Baylor repeated the question: "All he did was to prick your arm and hand with pins?"

"Yes."

"What did he conclude?"

"He concluded that I had impaired sensation and burning pains because the nerves had been cut during my radical surgery. He explained that many people who have dysathesia and causalgia— those are the medical names—cannot tolerate being touched in the affected area. That was why I couldn't bring myself to have intercourse with my husband, and why I was upset when my husband touched my body. The doctor was surprised that my surgeon didn't know this. He offered to testify on my behalf at the divorce trial.''

"Did you have any pain when he examined your arm?''

"No.''

"Did you have pain in the area of your chest where the radical mastectomy had been done and the wound had healed?''

"No.''

"That deep pain was gone?''

"Yes.''

"All you had when Dr. Engle examined you was this causalgia or dysathesia, as he called it?''

"Yes, and the shooting pain in my shoulder.''

"Now you and Dr. Engle seemed to get along pretty well together?''

"Yes.''

"He seemed to agree with you?''

"I didn't like him because he agreed with me, but because he explained certain medical phenomena so I could understand them. I respected him and knew I had met a physician who really was concerned about me.''

"Did you disagree on anything?'' Baylor persisted. He seemed to be trying to make a point.

"No, not that I can remember.''

"Did he render any further opinion about the medical profession generally?''

"Well, he did say the people who ran the American Medical Association, the head council, were a bunch of old men who didn't know what they were doing. This is all confidential. I assume you, as a lawyer, will keep this confidential,'' she added uneasily.

He answered her sharply, "I shall follow my duties as a lawyer defending my client in this case. All right?''

"I really don't know that I should be saying these things.'' She looked inquiringly at Mike.

"It's up to you and your lawyer. If you don't want to say anything, it is all right with me.''

Kathryn became angry. "Now you're contradicting yourself. You said you wanted me to tell you everything," she reminded him.

Baylor grew angry in turn. "I don't need any criticism from you, Mrs. Huffman. I get enough criticism at home."

Kathryn said firmly, "I will not say anything else about Dr. Engle."

"Are you refusing, therefore, to answer any further questions about your discussions with Dr. Engle?"

"Yes. I'm sorry I answered them to begin with."

Indignantly, Baylor demanded, "May we have a note at this point, please, so we can make a motion if necessary in court."

Mike Jefferson's temperature had been rising all through Baylor's interrogation of his client. He stood up. "Mr. Baylor, I don't know whether to apologize for my client's conduct or to complain to you that your remark was outrageous. Perhaps I should do both. Insofar as your conduct is concerned, Mr. Baylor, you can review the record at your leisure. The plaintiff will continue to answer any further questions that you have about Dr. Engle or anything else that you have in mind."

"Mr. Jefferson, first of all, I don't want you to apologize. Number two, I resent your comment that my remark was outrageous. Whatever was precipitated here was precipitated by your client's attitude. I resent your comment and ask that it be stricken from the record."

Baylor turned to Kathryn, and, trying hard to sound calm, he said, "Mrs. Huffman, we have reached a point in which we are asking about conversations that you had during the course of your treatment by Dr. Engle. You indicated before that he said something about the people in the AMA being old and so forth and I think I am getting now to the next point: did he or did he not ever say anything to you about whether this condition you had, the lump, the radical mastectomy, and so forth, was caused by The Pill?"

"No."

Baylor, his composure regained, continued, "Did he in later conversations indicate to you that he had done any reading on the subject of The Pill?"

"Only in relation to its possible effect on emotional illness and neurological impairment," replied Kathryn.

"Did you ever tell him that you had done any reading on the subject of The Pill?"

"Yes."

"Can you tell us the other books and articles you utilized to read up on The Pill in addition to what you have already read into the record?"

"Yes," Kathryn said, looking at Mike for an indication of whether or not she should go on.

However, Baylor went on quickly, "Will you be kind enough to either make a list of those or send your attorney copies of all the literature that you read on this subject so we may obtain copies, please?"

"Just a moment," Jefferson said. "Mrs. Huffman will do so if it is understood that the drug firm that is your client and the other defendants will furnish *us* with a bibliography of all related drug and medical research materials."

"Mr. Jefferson," retorted Baylor, "I don't think you have a right to put conditions on it. I want to know what this lady has read and if she will supply us with copies of what she has read. You can then proceed to get whatever information you want in the usual course."

"I think we will probably be able to comply with your request, Mr. Baylor," Mike answered. "However, we will request the same from all the defendants later on."

"Could we have some type of time limit, Mr. Jefferson—say, that we'll receive it from you in two weeks?"

"If you are going to get it without a motion, you will have it with the interrogatories, which should be within two weeks," responded Jefferson. "They will be sent to you in writing as you requested."

"It is understood on the record, Mr. Jefferson, that all of the literature which this lady has read on the subject will be given to us in her answers to the interrogatories, and if it does not there appear, we will then have to make a motion."

"Yes," replied Jefferson. "Let me add for the record that my client is facing further surgery, and it may be within the next several days. If, for any reason, she cannot give you the information you request in the interrogatories, I will indicate in the cover letter that it will be forthcoming."

"Now, Mrs. Huffman," Baylor said, turning back to her, "at this time can you remember other articles that you have read?"

"I remember the articles," Kathryn replied. "However, there have been hundreds. For example, there was one by Morton Mintz that I have here. . . ."

Mike took the article and handed it to Baylor, who glanced at it quickly and then handed it to the court reporter, instructing him to mark it for identification and place it on the record:

From the Record
The *Evening Record*, November 6, 1969*

A few days after the government learned that the artificial sweeteners called cyclamates caused bladder cancer in rats, it ordered an immediate halt to production of soft drinks and foods containing these chemicals.

But the oral contraceptives cause a wide variety of tumors in five species of experimental animals, including rats, and yet remain on sale with the blessing of the Department of Health, Education and Welfare.

The question for today is: Does this make any sense?

Dr. Herbert L. Ley, Jr., Commissioner of the Food and Drug Administration, told a news conference that

*Morton Mintz, *The Washington Post.*

the cyclamates, [now] classified as drugs, will be in a position entirely comparable to The Pill's position.

"The use of The Pill," he said, "is limited, the benefits are significant, and medical supervision is exercised."

A few weeks ago users of The Pill were estimated by the FDA's outside experts . . . to number 8.5 million in the United States and 10 million elsewhere. These figures excluded additional millions of women who have used The Pill but do so no longer.

This is limited use?

Dr. Ley termed the benefits significant. He didn't say for whom. He might, for example, get an argument from those women or their survivors who got a disabling or fatal blood clotting disease and who would not have taken The Pill had they been warned by their physicians or for that matter by the FDA about these and numerous other hazards.

In a 200-page report last month, the FDA's advisory committee said there is much data suggesting indirectly that steroid hormones such as those used in The Pill, particularly estrogen, may be carcinogenic—cancer-causing—in humans.

Most of the advisory committee's report is a catalogue of cause-effect relationships with The Pill that have been established, such as blood clotting, hair loss, skin blotching and liver disease, or suspected relationships that have not been established or disproved but are possibilities. In this category are not only cancer but also the effects on the offspring of users and on every organ system of the body.

. . . Dr. Roger O. Egeberg, the Assistant Secretary of HEW for health and scientific affairs, . . . said that the synthetic sweeteners had probably saved and prolonged a tremendous number of lives in the last few years by helping people to keep their weight down. . . .

There is no medical evidence that the cyclamates have saved lives. It turned out that there isn't even significant medical evidence that they help people keep their weight down. Dr. Egeberg finally conceded that his claim was based on nothing more than personal experience in losing 30 or 40 pounds after giving up cigarettes. . . .

Bringing his perspective to The Pill, Dr. Egeberg said that it has drawbacks. "But if you think of the number of young girls who are killed each year or were killed through aseptic abortion, you have something to balance there, too."

. . . Fatal blood clotting from The Pill kills about as many as die from criminal abortions.

Seriously misleading have been the pamphlets on The Pill prepared by the various makers and put by doctors in their waiting rooms, the points of sale. These booklets have touted The Pill in ways that at best understated the risks and at worst engaged in downright falsehood. One pamphlet, for example, claimed that the brand it was pushing had been proved safe. None has been proved safe.

What may be the most useful is to require the manufacturer to include in every package received by the user a fair, factual summary of the risks—in plain English. Of course, the FDA and organized medicine will oppose such an idea.

Chapter Six

"What did you read, Mrs. Huffman, that indicated to you that cancer of the breast had been caused by birth control pills?"

"That every species of animal given The Pill developed breast cancer."

"I am referring to human beings, not animals. Have you ever read any such articles?" Baylor asked in a put-down manner.

"I've read hundreds, and I've *heard* of many more. Eight months ago I heard Dr. Max Cutler testify before the Senate. He said it is relevant to transfer this animal data to man and that it must be regarded as significant. I was given a copy of his testimony at the hearing and I'd like it included for the record."

Mike handed the statement to the court reporter to mark for identification. In it, Dr. Cutler identified himself as the Medical Director of the Beverly Hills Cancer Research Foundation and a member of the surgical staffs of the Cedars of Lebanon and St. John's Hospitals in Los Angeles. He had been involved in cancer research and treatment for almost fifty years. He received his early training, beginning in 1924, at the Memorial Cancer Hospital in New York City, most of it under a Rockefeller Fellowship.

In 1931, Dr. Cutler founded the tumor clinic of the Michael Reese Hospital in Chicago, and was its director for five years. In 1936, he went under the auspices of the Rockefeller Foundation to

Peiping [Peking], China, as Visiting Professor of Surgery in the Medical College there. Two years later, he founded the Chicago Tumor Institute and served as its director for thirteen years. He has been consultant to the United States Veterans Administration, and a member of the National Advisory Cancer Council.

Dr. Cutler said at the hearings that the intimate relation between breast cancer and the ovaries has been known for a long time. When the ovaries are removed or treated with radiation, you see about forty percent remission in breast cancers in women under menopause age. This, he said, is because production of the hormone estrogen by the body is diminished after such treatment. In practice, he and his associates avoid using estrogens for fear of increasing the activity of an existing disease or stimulating the growth of latent centers of breast cancer. He explained that the incidence of cancer levels off after the age of fifty-five, and that it is higher in childless women than in women who bear children. A woman who has her first child under the age of twenty has considerable protection against breast cancer. All this shows a definite relation between ovarian activity and breast cancer.

"The tissues of the breast present a highly sensitive target for the ovarian hormones and have a great potential for the development of cancer," he said. "The early detection of breast cancer often presents formidable difficulties. Not infrequently when a lump is first felt, either by the patient or by her physician, she is already in a relatively advanced stage of cancer. . . ."

Then he turned his attention to The Pill. "The difficulty of demonstrating a causative relationship between the oral contraceptives and breast cancer obviously relates to the long latent period between exposure and final effect. A minimum of ten years is required before reliable results can be expected. Unfortunately, this experiment upon millions of women might prove to be too costly to contemplate."

Dr. Cutler concluded by saying that the question has arisen as to whether the benefits outweigh the risks. "The women who have been taking The Pill for five years or more are too few and too young to demonstrate any changes with respect to the risks of increasing the incidence of breast cancer. That risk is a potential time bomb with a fuse at least fifteen to twenty years in length. I share the hope that the concern about this danger may be unfounded, and that the considerable experimental evidence may be inapplicable to women, but this is a gamble which is difficult to justify because of the large numbers of women at risk.''

Kathryn put down the paper and went on. ''An article in the *British Medical Journal* tells that a doctor found a definite causation between the birth control pill and breast cancer in some of his patients. He felt the cancer risk might overshadow any other disorder caused by The Pill, including blood clots.'' She picked up the article. ''He says, 'It is striking that the possible induction of carcinoma is barely mentioned in the countless discussions on The Pill that can be read in the non-medical press. Have the sociologists (and the drug houses) won the argument yet again before the problem has been properly formulated, let alone solved?' ''

Mike Jefferson took the article from Kathryn and handed it to the court reporter.

Baylor looked over his notes and looked slowly up at Kathryn. ''Now let's go back to your arm, please, your left arm. You noticed a swelling there in January of 1970?''

''That's correct.''

''Who has been treating you for that condition since that date? Has anyone?''

''Well, as I said, Dr. Engle suggested I should see Dr. Buchanan. His report has been placed in the record.''

From the Record
June 29, 1970
Huffman, Kathryn #72194

This twenty-four-year-old woman entered Cliffs Hospital to have a surgical removal of the ovaries to effect a diminution of estrogen productivity, as she has an estrogen-dependent medullary cancer with lymphoid infiltration which was first diagnosed on November 18, 1968.

On June 17, 1970, a surgical excision of the left supraclavicular lymph nodes showed metastasis to the regional lymph nodes. I advised the patient that she had less than six months to live but might extend this period if the ovaries were removed. . . .

Robert Buchanan, M.D.

"Is Dr. Buchanan presently treating you for the arm?" Baylor continued.

"No, Dr. Herman Doenitz is presently treating me for my arm. Dr. Doenitz is a cancer internist."

"What is he doing for your arm?"

"He can't do anything to reduce the swelling. He prescribes medication for the pain."

"Has the pain gotten worse?"

"It has been about the same for the last two months."

"What did Dr. Doenitz say is wrong with your arm?"

"He feels there might be a tumor blocking the circulation and pressing on a nerve. He wants me to go to Memorial Hospital in New York next week for surgery to determine the nature of the tumor and what, if anything, can be done about it."

"Did you ask Dr. Doenitz whether or not there was any relation between your condition and the things that have happened to you?"

"Yes. Dr. Doenitz believes that cancer cells were spread to my shoulder and my armpit when I had the radical mastectomy."

"Are you implying that this happened *as a result of* the radical mastectomy?"

"Yes. That's the impression I got. I didn't pursue it with him."

"Have you asked him whether or not there is any connection between this condition you have just described and your having taken the pills, the birth control pills?"

"I don't recall asking him that. I haven't asked for his opinion about The Pill and breast cancer. I am too anxious to have him as a doctor who will be able to help me, rather than as a doctor who might be afraid of getting involved in a lawsuit. No, I haven't pursued this subject with him."

"Is Dr. Doenitz going to operate on you next week?"

"No. Dr. Philip Hakon will operate on me."

"Another doctor! Who is Dr. Philip Hakon?"

"He's a surgeon at Memorial Hospital who was recommended by Dr. Doenitz."

"Have you seen him?"

"Yes, I saw him last week."

"Have you talked to this doctor about whether The Pill could be causatively connected with your condition?"

"No."

Baylor stopped long enough to look over some notes he held in his hand. The long questioning was clearly taking its toll on Kathryn.

"Now, let's go back to Dr. Buchanan. He performed some type of operative procedure on you?"

"Yes."

"Would you repeat for the record what he did to you?"

It was obvious that Kathryn was fighting off great pain and trying to get a grip on herself as she answered, "First, he removed a lymph node near my left collarbone. He. . . ."

"How do you feel at the present time?" Baylor asked, cutting her off.

Kathryn repeated his question, "How do I feel?"

"Yes," he said flatly.

"How do you mean? Emotionally or physically?"

"Any way you want to tell us," he replied with a shrug.

"I don't feel very well," Kathryn replied slowly.

"Do you have pain at the present time?"

"Yes, I do," Kathryn declared. It was evident that she was trying not to display the extent of her pain.

"In what parts of your body?"

"In my hand."

"The left hand?"

"My left hand."

"Do you have any other pain or discomfort in any other parts of your body?"

She could not conceal her suffering. Beaded perspiration appeared on her forehead. "I have sharp shooting pains in my shoulder," she answered.

"Does the pain come and go?"

"Yes. It's a cyclical kind of pain that goes from my hand to my shoulder," she replied. She rubbed her left arm with her other hand.

"Do you have any other kind of pain?"

"No, just the grabbing, sharp pain all through my arm, that comes and goes."

"Do you have any other pain right now? You asked before about physical and mental. I think you said emotional," Baylor prompted her.

"Yes, I do," she replied, taking a deep breath.

Baylor's glasses were in his hand again, and as he looked at the other lawyers he said in an unconcerned, matter-of-fact tone, "Do you want to tell us how you feel emotionally?"

"Emotionally?" Kathryn repeated. "I'll tell you, Mr. Baylor. You probably saved my life last night, or prolonged it, whatever. I would have killed myself if it weren't that I was going to appear here for the deposition today. That's the one thing that is keeping me alive. The pain is so terrible, so excruciating, that I couldn't take it if I didn't have something this important to stay alive for. I can tell you're trying to upset me, by the way you are examining me. You'd like to bury me with all the rest of the truth about birth control pills but actually, you're keeping me alive."

Baylor stood up. "Mrs. Huffman. . . ."

"You are keeping me alive!" she repeated. "I am going to stay alive, at least long enough to complete this deposition, no matter how much pain I have!" Kathryn declared.

"I move to have those remarks stricken!" Dr. Lawrence's lawyer shouted.

Baylor appeared stunned. His face was pale and his voice trembled as he slowly said, "Mrs. Huffman, I have no feeling one way or the other except that you are a litigant and I am trying to do my job."

Kathryn gave him an angry look. "You're trying to upset me by harassing me. It's obvious you have no feeling."

Visibly shaken, he protested, "No, I am *not* trying to harass you. The record may show that you are not the only one in this room that had cancer. I had it myself, if you want to get personal, which we shouldn't. I want it on the record that I am not trying to upset you. I don't think you should make those remarks."

"Did *your* physician prescribe medication that triggered your cancer, or possibly caused it, as my physicians did, Mr. Baylor?"

Baylor stared at her, but did not reply.

"I know that you feel you are doing your job as the defendants' lawyer, and that means confronting me, the plaintiff. But the record will show that you have harassed me all through this deposition," Kathryn said hotly. "I might not be alive when the judge reviews this record, Mr. Baylor, but I know he will agree with me and let the record stand. I'm going to win this case, to save other women from what happened to me. I'm fighting you and your clients and horrible pain and *death* to get a change in the way medicine and drugs are handed out. I'm going to show the harm that medical technology can cause by prescribing unnecessary, harmful drugs, and I'm not going to die until I do!"

Everyone in the room was still.

Baylor bowed his head, looked down at the table covered with papers and in a voice scarcely above a whisper, said, "I move the whole thing should be stricken from the record—her comments and mine, both."

"I suggest we don't strike *anything* from the record!" Mike said. "I do think Mr. Baylor is correct, to a certain extent. I needn't tell you my client is desperately ill. Kathryn, try to answer the questions without referring to Mr. Baylor. Mr. Baylor and the other attorneys are doing a job. And, in case you don't know it, everyone in this room has to get somewhat emotionally involved because of what is happening to you. Nobody wants to harass you. Everyone here is doing a job for their clients as we all are sworn to do. If the question is put to you again in terms of your emotional situation, answer the question without making any specific reference to Mr. Baylor. The rest of the material, if this is part of your emotional picture, belongs on the record.''

Dr. Lawrence's lawyer, Mr. Arnold, spoke. ''I move that it be stricken.''

''I want to have it noted whether or not counsel will exclude from the record all this conversation,'' said Mr. Griffiths, who represented the other drug company. ''I suggest it be removed.''

''I suggest it be removed as well,'' Baylor added quietly as he looked down at the floor.

''I agree,'' Dr. Canaris' lawyer said.

''How do you feel about it?'' Griffiths asked Mike.

''I don't know what we are going to do later on; maybe I can join in that later. Let's proceed. There have been several objections made by some of us to strike portions of the record and I would be perfectly willing to consider that at a later point. I'd like to see the whole record before we take any steps such as that,'' Mike replied.

A somewhat subdued Baylor resumed his examination of Kathryn, ''We were trying to find out your emotional state and you told us that you were going to win this case and you stayed awake because you were coming here today.''

She corrected him, ''I stayed alive.''

''All right,'' he said, obviously annoyed. This damaging statement was now a matter of record. ''Let's hear the rest of it.''

Kathryn drank some water and thought for a moment about the question put to her before answering, ''What I said before sums it up pretty well.''

''You took medication last night, didn't you?'' Baylor asked, taking a different tack.

"Yes."

"What was the purpose of that medication?"

"To allow me to sleep. I also take pain medication."

"What is the medication? Do you know the name of it?" Baylor demanded.

"Yes. The sleeping medication is called Tuinal, T-u-i-n-a-l. I take nine grains every night in addition to Amytal, to enhance the effect of the Tuinal."

"Under whose supervision are you taking this medication?" Baylor continued, slowly regaining his composure.

"The sleeping medication I'm taking under Dr. Engle's supervision. Dr. Doenitz prescribes my pain medication. I take one Percodan every three hours. When necessary, I take Demerol, if I can't wait out the three hours. At times, it's necessary for either my father or mother to give me an injection of Demerol during the night. I also take Numorphan. . . ."

"Your parents give you injections?" Baylor interrupted her, raising his eyebrows.

"As needed. Dr. Doenitz authorized them to do so," Kathryn replied.

"Would you mind telling us, generally speaking, what your complaints have been to Dr. Engle between April and July of 1970? What have you told him has been bothering you, please?" Baylor asked.

"The pain."

"Anything else?"

"Not really. The whole thing has been an effort to relieve me of excruciating pain. He can't do anything about the cancer."

"Are you telling us your complaint to Dr. Engle has been about the pain in your left arm area? Is that what you are telling us?"

"Yes."

"Nothing else. Is that right?"

"We might stray into a conversation about something and I couldn't begin to remember all the things we have talked about, but it always centers around the idea of pain."

"You have your arm in a sling," Baylor said.

"Yes. That was recommended by Dr. Doenitz."

"For what reason?"

"When a person has a radical mastectomy, often they try to improve the circulation by wrapping the arm in an elastic bandage, which pushes the blood up. That's part of the problem. The blood can't circulate properly. I think it helps the pain a little bit, but it doesn't really do much good. The sling is just to make it easier for me to carry the weight of my arm."

Mr. Baylor closed the notebook in front of him, took off his glasses and rubbed his eyes. "I have no further questions." He motioned to Mr. Griffiths.

Chapter Seven

Later in the day, November 3, 1970.

Griffiths was a rather short, stocky man with receding red hair. He was dressed with a flair toward the latest in men's fashions. His suit was dark green and he wore an apple green shirt with a harmonizing tie.

He introduced himself to Kathryn. "I am Charles Griffiths, as you may remember, and I represent the Lears Pharmaceutical Corporation, manufacturer of Mordrine Birth Control Pills.

"Mrs. Huffman, has any doctor that you have seen for treatment, or any doctor with whom you have been in consultation, or, in fact, any doctor that you have had any conversation with relating to this breast cancer that resulted in the removal of the left breast—has any one of them ever told you that The Pill, the birth control pill, was in any way the cause of this cancer that was found in your left breast?"

"Objection!" shouted Mike. He motioned to Kathryn to remain silent. "The witness is instructed not to answer the question. I consider that not to be a question."

"This is a conversation," replied Griffiths.

"Well," said Mike, "the material has been covered. You are working out your summation."

Griffiths snapped, "I am asking a question. I want to know the names of those doctors who told her that The Pill caused her cancer!"

"I think in view of the very exhaustive manner in which Mr. Baylor has covered every single physician. . . ." Mike interjected.

Griffiths cut him off. "Am I going to be precluded by Mr. Baylor's examination?"

Baylor joined in. "I don't think it was exhaustive. I just got tired. I don't think that is a legitimate objection to Mr. Griffiths' question."

Mike was immovable. "I will instruct the witness not to answer the question."

"I think you ought to make a motion," said Baylor to Griffiths.

"The court may not back me up," said Mike Jefferson, "but I think I'm right."

Legal wrangling continued among the four lawyers for a considerable length of time. Kathryn rotated her shoulders and pulled back on them to relieve the pain a bit. She took a deep breath of the smoke-filled air and started to cough. No one seemed aware of her discomfort as she took a sip of water.

Her eyes fell on a nautical clock that was centered on the wall facing her. The deposition had taken her back in time but the clock's hands continued forward. Time was running out.

As Kathryn watched the lawyers wrangling, trying to keep her remarks off the record, she thought back over the terrifying experiences she had had since she first felt the lump on her breast.

As horrifying as it was to have her breast cut off, she felt having her ovaries removed had snuffed out the last bit of life she had in her. True, she wanted a professional career. Perhaps she would have practiced law at The Hague or worked in diplomatic circles— but that would be after she had had her children. Above all, she had wanted to have children. . . .

Griffiths' voice caught her attention.

"For the record, then, in view of counsel's directing his client not to answer the question I have asked, I have no alternative but to make a motion to the court for a ruling on these questions, and I will therefore terminate my cross-examination until the court rules on the matter.''

"As far as I am concerned,'' Mike casually replied, "the rules will control on that. I think they cover it very completely.''

"I don't know anything about the rules,'' Griffiths said curtly, "but I want my statement on the record!''

With an air of finality, Mike said, "It appears that the second deposition has reached an impasse until the court rules as to whether you are right or I am right on this issue. Therefore, I shall bid you gentlemen a good day.''

Mike had warned Kathryn about the strain the deposition would place on her emotionally and physically. He knew how painful it would be for her to go back over her experiences with eighteen doctors, time after time—experiences that most people try to forget. But Kathryn wasn't that kind of person. She had written a letter to Mike in answer to his warning:

> If I must die . . . and die so terribly. . . , at least let me die feeling fulfilled. I want to feel I've done everything I could to expose this secrecy of silence that exists about The Pill. I want to warn others, so they won't be misinformed or have to suffer the pain and agony I've had. . . .

Chapter Eight

November 11, 1970.

Huffman, Kathryn Stuart
Memorial Hospital #102216

This 25-year-old woman was admitted to Memorial Hospital for surgical incision of the left regional lymph nodes to determine whether radiation is the treatment of choice. A needle aspiration biopsy was made of the mass which was malignant.

Following surgery we had a discussion with Dr. Doenitz of Chemotherapy and Dr. Hastings of Radiation Therapy. Whereas an intensive course of chemotherapy was recommended, the patient refused to be hospitalized at this time for an extensive period due to pending court proceedings. Therefore, she will undergo radiation therapy again. The skeletal survey, liver scan and brain scan were negative.

Prognosis: Terminal   Estimated 3-4 months.

November 12, 1970.

Before being discharged from Memorial Hospital, Kathryn was taken to the cashier's window to pay her bill. She was accompanied by her mother.

"$990.45! Mother, can you believe that! I was only here for a few days, in a small room with four other patients, and the bill is almost a thousand dollars! And that doesn't even include the surgeon's fee . . . !" Kathryn's bills so far were over twenty thousand dollars. "I must be living in Samuel Butler's *Erewhon*," she said bitterly, "where the sick are punished and fined for being ill and then are condemned to die."

December 9, 1970.

Huffman, Kathryn Stuart
Memorial Hospital #102216
The patient completed the second series of 16 cobalt treatments which extended from November 17, 1970, to December 9, 1970, on an out-patient basis at the office of Dr. Norman Hastings.

December 30, 1970.

Huffman, Kathryn Stuart
The Rehabilitation Institute #121998
Physical therapy has been initiated in an attempt to enable the patient to regain some use of her left hand and arm which have become "frozen" and badly swollen due to terminal cancer.

Noon. January 16, 1971, Mike Jefferson's office.

It was a brisk winter's day. The sun hung high in the sky, too far away to warm the throngs of people scurrying below. Overcoats were buttoned up, and men held on to their hats. Collars were raised in an effort to cover the chins of kerchief-clad women. People hurried across the street, ignoring the traffic lights.

Kathryn paused a moment in front of the window to watch them before taking her seat between her mother and Mike. Mike touched her hand as she sat down. The sound of a man's voice saying her name brought her back to reality.

The court reporter recited: "Kathryn Stuart Huffman, the plaintiff, having been duly sworn according to law by the officer, testifies as follows. Direct examination by Mr. Griffiths."

"Mrs. Huffman, I am Charles Griffiths. I represent Lears Pharmaceutical Company, the company that produces the contraceptive pill Mordrine. Last time, I think we ended on the question as to whether you had ever received a written or oral report from any doctor that set up a causative relationship between the contraceptive pills and the cancerous condition that led to the removal of your breast. There was a hearing on that motion, and as a result, the court confined the question to those doctors set forth by you in answers to the interrogatories that Mr. Baylor's office propounded on behalf of the contraceptive pill 'Cycle . . .' what?"

" . . . mide," Baylor supplied, "Cyclemide."

"Now then," Griffiths continued, "can you recall all the doctors whose names were set forth by you in answer to these interrogatories?"

"Yes, of course," Kathryn replied.

"Now, as to any of those doctors that are set forth in answer to your interrogatories, have you or anyone on your behalf ever received any oral or written report alleging a causative relationship between either of these contraceptive pills and the breast cancer which was removed in your case?" Griffiths asked without taking a breath.

Kathryn looked at him in disbelief. It was as if they had never left that room in Mike's office, even though two and one-half months had elapsed between that time and this.

Everything was going backwards again as she heard Mike say, "Don't answer the question, Mrs. Huffman." In a patient voice, he reminded the attorney, "Mr. Griffiths, I think either you or I misunderstood the court's order. I think we sent you a copy of it. The application that you made was denied."

"That's right. You sent me the order," replied Griffiths. "Go ahead, Mr. Jefferson, make your point."

"Where is the copy of the order?" Baylor demanded. He stood up suddenly and attempted to grab the papers from Griffiths' hand. "If I may?" he said.

Griffiths held the papers over his head so Baylor could not reach them, saying, "The order merely says the two questions propounded. . . ."

Baylor interrupted, "I don't have a copy of the order."

". . . were denied," abruptly added Griffiths, ignoring Baylor entirely.

"Let's get off the record," Mike interjected, annoyed by the bickering.

Griffiths glared at Mike and replied, "Let's stay on the record."

Baylor shouted, "I would like at this time to throw a monkey wrench into these proceedings. I would like an answer to that question."

"I'll ask you the exact same question by way of interrogatories, if that's what you want, Mr. Jefferson," threatened Griffiths. "Now, then, Mrs. Huffman," Griffiths asked finally, turning to Kathryn, "can you recall when it was that you first had occasion to talk to any doctor about a prescription of contraceptive pills for yourself; when was it?"

Kathryn was quite pale today. Her skin had a waxen-white beauty, far from the youthful, pink cheeks she had once had—only a few months ago. Now it seemed to just barely cover her cheekbones. Her warm brown eyes seemed more deeply set because of the bluish darkness encircling them. But she was as poised as ever. Not showing any pain, she replied, "It was on April the 11th, 1968 that I saw Dr. Lawrence to discuss birth control methods."

Griffiths unexpectedly placed his papers on the table and said, "Thank you, Mrs. Huffman, I have no further questions at this time."

The next lawyer approached her. He was carefully, almost over-carefully fashionably dressed.

"Mrs. Huffman, I represent Dr. Lawrence. My name is Harold Arnold. I just want to ask you a few questions. When you discovered this cyst or lump in your breast, you had never noticed it there before, is that correct?"

"That's correct."

"And this was about two or three weeks after you started taking a birth control pill other than the one Dr. Lawrence prescribed originally?"

"Yes."

"Did you stop taking the birth control pill when you noticed this lump or cyst?"

"No, I didn't."

"Did you go back to see Dr. Canaris who prescribed the other birth control pill?"

"No, I didn't."

"When you went to Dr. Lawrence on September 6, 1968, and informed him you had a lump on your breast, I understand that he told you to discontinue the birth control pills?"

"Yes, that's right."

"And did you discontinue them?"

"Yes."

"And he wanted you to see him again in one month, did he not?"

"Yes."

"He also indicated to you that he wanted you to go through one more period and at the end of that time to check you. Is that correct?"

"No. He didn't say anything about waiting for my period before seeing him. He said to make an appointment when he got back from his vacation. That he'd be gone for about one month."

"When did you get an appointment?"

"October 10, 1968."

"From September 6th to October 10th, I take it, you took no further birth control pills of any kind?"

"That's right."

"When you went back on October 10th, 1968, Dr. Lawrence examined you. He recommended or suggested that the lump be excised, did he not?"

"No. He said that there were a number of different things that could be done regarding the lump."

"What did he tell you?"

"He said one thing they could do would be to drain the lump, to let the fluid out and thereby shrink it. Or it could be excised—cut out. Or I might wait to see if it would shrink. He said if I wanted the lump to be excised, he would recommend Dr. Ivan Frederick. He didn't particularly push for any one of these methods. He left that decision up to me."

"With respect to the suggestion of the excision, did he give you Dr. Frederick's name and address?"

"Yes."

"And did you call Dr. Frederick?"

"Yes, and I went to see him."

"When did you go to see him?"

"I don't know the exact date. It was in October."

"When you went there, Dr. Frederick examined your breast, did he not?"

"Yes."

"He detected the cyst or lump that you had?"

"Yes."

"What was his recommendation?"

"He felt the lump should be excised."

"This is where the controversy developed about your signing an authorization?"

"Yes."

"And then you went to see Dr. Mark Halsey at Barnard Hospital in New York?"

"Yes. And he was not as adamant as Dr. Frederick that it should be excised. He said to me, 'You can let it alone or you can have it excised. It really doesn't matter.' He was passive about it. I felt I needed another surgeon's opinion at that point."

"That is when you went to Dr. Julius Wilkinson?"

"Yes."

"Now, Dr. Frederick didn't lead you to believe there was any critical problem that meant you should have the operation immediately, did he?"

"No."

"Did Dr. Halsey at Barnard share the same view that there was no urgency in having the operation—that it was not an emergency?"

"Yes. Even more so."

"Now, did you ever consult a Dr. Thomas Lewis?"

"No."

"Did you ever speak with a Dr. Thomas Lewis?"

"Yes."

"Where did you meet him and when did you meet him?"

"Approximately in the spring of 1970 in my lawyer's office."

"Is Dr. Lewis a lawyer?"

"He is a physician and a lawyer."

"How did you come to meet Dr. Lewis?"

"He was associated with one of my lawyers, Mr. Paul Slater."

"Did you subsequently retain Mr. Slater or his firm in respect to this case?"

"Yes."

"And in connection with that, is that where you met Dr. Lewis?"

"Yes."

"You did not see Dr. Lewis for any treatment, did you?"

"No."

"He only spoke to you as a lawyer?"

"Yes."

"A lawyer with a medical degree, is that right?"

"Yes."

"Now, did Mr. Slater or Dr. Lewis send you to any doctors in New York for examination?"

"No."

"Did they send you to any doctors anywhere for examination?"

"No."

"Did they recommend that you see any doctors?"

"No."

"Did they recommend that you retain any doctors or that they would retain doctors in connection with your case?"

"Well, we spoke of the importance of getting expert medical points of view about the case and they said that they would work on that."

"Did you authorize them to retain somebody?"

"Let me interrupt at this point," said Mike Jefferson. "I think you've gone over the line now, Mr. Arnold. I wasn't sure you really intended to, but apparently you did. So, I'll have to instruct the witness not to answer questions relating to her conversations with her attorneys."

Arnold nodded and continued, "Mrs. Huffman, have you conferred with any medical doctors other than the ones who have treated you?"

"Yes."

"Dr. Lawrence had been your family doctor for some period of time, had he not?"

"Yes."

"And he examined you on an annual basis when you went for your checkup?"

"That's right."

"And various problems that developed during your lifetime from the age twelve up to the time you saw him for contraceptive prescriptions?"

"That's correct."

"Incidently, when you talked to him about birth control, did you tell him your husband's vehement, irrevocable refusal to use any equipment of any kind himself—that he wanted you to take the precautions?"

"I told him that my husband wanted me to use the birth control pill."

"And that he didn't want to use anything himself?"

"I don't know how much of the discussion I related to Dr. Lawrence other than to say my husband wanted me to take The

Pill. I didn't say, 'Don't tell me that my husband should use something.' I left it wide open."

"Incidentally, what doctors are you seeing now?"

"Dr. Herman Doenitz. He is a cancer internist and—"

"How often do you see Dr. Doenitz?" Arnold interrupted.

"About every ten days."

"Does he check you out and follow through with you?"

"Yes."

"Does he prescribe medication?"

"Yes. He prescribes medication for my pain."

"What medication are you on at the moment from Dr. Doenitz?"

"Percodan, Demerol and Numorphan."

"Do you see any other doctor?"

"Yes. Dr. Alvin Engle."

"How frequently do you see him?"

"About once every two weeks."

"He is a psychiatrist?"

"He's a neuropsychiatrist," Kathryn corrected him.

"Does he prescribe any medication for you?"

"Yes. Tuinal, so I can sleep at night."

"Any other doctors at the moment?"

"No."

"Are you working?"

"I'm trying to complete my doctorate before. . . ." Kathryn looked down at her papers and shook her head, unable to continue her sentence.

"Before—?" Arnold said, encouraging her to go on.

Kathryn looked at him intently and shook her head from side to side. "Nothing," she said.

"Please finish your response," he demanded.

"Before I die," she answered quietly.

There was complete silence. Then Baylor shouted, "I move that be stricken from the record."

Arnold fumbled with his glasses to regain his composure.

"What is the status of your divorce proceeding in New York?" he asked finally.

"We're about to begin the divorce trial."

"Thank you, Mrs. Huffman," he said and sat down.

The next attorney approached Kathryn. A tall, well-built man, his black hair with graying sideburns and the gray streak in front made him look distinguished.

"Mrs. Huffman," he began, "My name is Bernard Ressler and I represent Dr. Vittorio Canaris. You testified during the previous depositions that you had read articles, particularly in *The New York Times*, that caused you some concern. They made you think that there might be some danger connected with the birth control pill. Is that correct?"

"Yes."

"What specifically did these articles warn of as a possible result of using the birth control pill?"

"Well, the article in *The Times* that I referred to when I spoke to Dr. Lawrence discussed thrombophlebitis, blood clots, and said there was definitely a relationship. The *Good Housekeeping* article was very broad. It just talked about possible dangers because The Pill was new. The oral contraceptive is still experimental in a sense, it said, and no one knows all the possible diseases or problems that might develop."

"If you can, I'd like you to go through all the conversations that you had with Dr. Canaris. Tell us everything that happened during that visit with Dr. Canaris."

"Well, the very first thing that happened was he gave me a physical examination before talking to me. He examined me internally and examined my breasts."

"After the physical examination, what conversation took place?"

"I went into his office and the first thing I recall him saying to me was that I was very tight, nervous. He said something to the effect that everything seemed to be okay. He said he would let me know later about the Pap test. He wanted to know what I used as a birth control measure.''

"In other words, he brought up the birth control measure for the first time?''

"I believe so. I said I was using Cyclemide pills. He said he had a lot of patients on the birth control pill and he never heard anybody complain as I had complained about it. He suggested that perhaps the reason I was complaining about so many side effects was that I was dubious about taking The Pill and these side effects in fact were a product of my imagination, rather than really caused by The Pill. He said, 'Maybe you'll feel better if I change the brand,' so he changed the brand to Mordrine. I took the new prescription and had it filled.''

"You took this new prescription for a period of about one month, is that right?''

"For one month.''

"When did the lump appear in your breast, first show up, as close as you can pinpoint it?''

"As I said, I have to guess somewhere between the 20th and 30th of August. It was two or three weeks after I saw Dr. Canaris.''

"When did your confidence in Dr. Canaris disappear?''

"During the office visit when he said I was imagining the side effects from the birth control pill. And then he assumed I was frigid with my husband because I was 'up-tight' during the internal examination.''

"As a matter of fact, you were pretty mad about that, weren't you?''

Kathryn's face reddened as she recalled Dr. Canaris' insolence and she replied, "I was furious!''

"Did you ever call Dr. Canaris and tell him that you had found a lump in your breast?''

"No. I didn't want to have anything more to do with Dr. Canaris.''

"How about any correspondence with him?"

"I wrote a letter to him before the lump appeared, saying that the side effects were going away. I thought he might be interested in knowing that."

"At the time you wrote this letter, the lump had not appeared, is that correct?"

"Yes."

"Now, Mrs. Huffman," he went on, glancing at the letter, "in the second paragraph you make reference to the fact that you consulted with another physician. Would you tell us who this other physician was and what the circumstances were of the consultation?"

"As I said before, I was very upset after seeing Dr. Canaris." Kathryn took a long breath. "One of my family's dearest and closest friends is a psychiatrist, Dr. Beatrice Woods. I wrote her a letter telling her what had happened and asked for her opinion. Her husband, Dr. Seymour Woods, is a surgeon, and they phoned me as soon as they got my letter. They felt my side effects were in fact real. They had many patients who experienced the side effects that I had been describing. They said Mordrine was less concentrated than Cyclemide and that's why I felt less ill from that pill. They did not approve of the birth control pill *per se*, although I had not discussed this matter with them before I started taking The Pill. I had tried to remain as objective and fair as possible, by only consulting physicians who were not personal friends."

Ressler said quickly, "That is all I have," and sat down.

"I believe it's my turn now," Mike said.

Ressler waved his index finger at Mike. "All right, go ahead."

Mike looked directly at his client and addressed her in a gentle manner. "Mrs. Huffman, as your lawyer, I am going to cross-examine you, and I would like to start at the beginning of the deposition, when Mr. Baylor began examining you. Should we start now or would you rather wait until you feel better?"

"I think we had better start now."

"My question, Mrs. Huffman, is to what extent in your discussions with Dr. Lawrence was there any reference to dangers about taking The Pill?"

"I said, 'Dr. Lawrence, is it safe for me to take The Pill? Would I have any serious ill effects from taking The Pill other than the side effects you mentioned—nausea, sore breasts and headaches?' He said I would not."

"He told you it was safe?"

"Yes. He said I might get side effects that would make me feel uncomfortable for a short time. But my body would adjust and I wouldn't get sick from them or get serious ill effects from taking The Pill. I believed him!"

"Was there any discussion with Dr. Canaris as to whether or not there were dangers in using The Pill?"

"Yes. The discussion was along the exact same lines that I had with Dr. Lawrence. I asked him about the safety of The Pill so far as my health was concerned. He said it was absolutely safe."

Mike Jefferson looked at his notes and asked, "Would you tell us what pain you felt after surgery? The surgery that occurred on November 18 and 20, 1968."

"The pain was intense. I was bleeding profusely from my chest. I had to walk doubled over. The surgeon and the nurses kept forcing me to exercise my arm, and that was terribly painful. The pain was just practically intolerable!"

"Were you at this time having any difficulty in sleeping?"

"Yes. I couldn't sleep well without taking Tuinals, which are barbiturates."

"How long did the pain continue at that level?"

"It continued at that level for about two months after the surgery—through January, I would say. Then I went back to school, to the University."

"Once you began your studies, were you able to continue through 1969 without any recurrence of the pain?"

While Kathryn was trying to remember how she felt in February, 1969, Baylor commented, "While the lady is thinking of her answer, I'd like to object to the leading character of your questions, particularly in view of the peculiar circumstances of this case."

"Let me rephrase the question, Mrs. Huffman," Mike said without looking at Baylor. "Would you tell us what the course of your condition was insofar as the pain, if any, that you had in 1969? Did you have more pain after February, 1969?"

She tried to be precise in her answer. "It's hard to separate the physical pain I had from the mental anguish I was going through, Mr. Jefferson. The wound refused to heal, and that was distressing for me both physically and emotionally. I had to change the dressing every night. I had to see the blood flowing from the hole in my chest where my breast had been. When I lay down to sleep, I had to lie on my back. I felt a very heavy pressure on my chest that was eventually diagnosed as dysathesia."

Mike paused and looked from her to the papers he was holding. "Mrs. Huffman, if you recall, Mr. Baylor, defense attorney for one of the drug firms, asked you why you were so concerned about a scar that would be on an area nobody would see except your husband and you. You replied, 'I thought it would be disfiguring.' He asked, 'Is that what was bothering you?' You replied, 'Yes.' Mr. Baylor continued, 'I don't suppose your relation with your husband, getting along as man and wife, in any way had you upset or nervous at all?' You replied, 'I thought I might be less attractive to my husband after surgery.' Would you accept the proposition that your concern about being disfigured was due only to your concern about your relationship with your husband?"

"No."

"Would you care to elaborate on this point?"

"Breasts have been made very important in our culture, and I can't escape being influenced by that. They just about decide whether or not a woman is desirable. I can't be emotionally detached about them: they're a very significant part of my body, and I can't think of them as separate from me, any more than a man could think of his sexual organs as separate if they were deformed —let alone cut off.''

''I object and make a motion that these remarks be stricken from the record,'' Baylor said.

''Mr. Baylor, I am only clarifying an issue you previously raised,'' Mike explained. ''Mrs. Huffman, would you tell us what the course of your condition was insofar as the pain you had, if any, in 1970?''

''I had undergone a lot of personal suffering as well as pain from what Dr. Engle describes as a causalgia.''

''What is causalgia?'' Mike asked.

''Has the lady finished her answer?'' Baylor queried. ''If so, I want to make a motion to strike the answer as not responsive to the question. If she's not finished, I shall wait. If she is, the motion is on record.''

''Go ahead,'' Mike said to Kathryn with a nod of reassurance.

''Causalgia is supposed to be a severe form of pain, a burning pain, affecting the nervous system. I was in a great deal of pain both physically and mentally.''

''What physician did you consult in April of 1970 regarding the pain in your left shoulder?'' asked Mike.

''We had already been to several doctors who specialized in breast cancer and they were unable to help me. So we decided to try a neurologist for the pain and I saw Dr. Engle in April of 1970.''

''When did he make his diagnosis, if you recall, of causalgia due to surgery?''

''That diagnosis. . . .''

Baylor interrupted, ''Where is the fact upon which that question is predicated?''

''I wanted to object to that also, Mr. Jefferson,'' added Arnold.

''I object to the form,'' added Griffiths.

''I'll rephrase the question,'' Mike said. ''In your answers to interrogatories, Mrs. Huffman, you refer to that diagnosis by Dr.

Engle. When did Dr. Engle first tell you of the diagnosis of causalgia?''

"I object to it as to form," shouted Griffiths.

"I object to that," Arnold declared.

"I object to it also," Baylor echoed.

"You can't get it this way," Arnold said in a warning voice to Mike.

"I believe the record shows that Mrs. Huffman has already testified that Dr. Engle told her she had causalgia. Am I incorrect in that?" Mike asked of the group as a whole.

"I object to any conversation between her and Dr. Engle," said Baylor in a bored voice.

"I object to it too, Mr. Jefferson; you can't do it this way," Arnold warned.

Another legal wrangle developed. The attorneys argued for several minutes. Finally Mike turned to Kathryn and smiled encouragingly at her. "Go ahead," he said.

Disregarding the hostility in the atmosphere, and despite the fact that she seemed ready to faint, Kathryn answered, "It was in September of 1970."

"What treatment has Dr. Engle given you?" Mike asked, pushing ahead through all the objections being raised by the defendants' lawyers.

Baylor was determined not to let her continue. "I think the record should show that this information is available to the plaintiff's attorney through other sources and it should enhance our objection to the form and substance of your inquiry, Mr. Jefferson."

"What treatment has Dr. Engle given you?" Mike asked Kathryn.

"There is no treatment that you can give. . . ." she began, but Baylor again cut her off.

"I ask that be stricken as not being responsive," he said.

"Go on, Kathryn," Mike told her, ignoring Baylor's objection.

She sighed deeply and started again to speak. "According to Dr.

Engle, there is nothing you can do for causalgia. You just have to wait for it to go away, if it ever will. He tried a nerve block, but it was not successful. He referred me to Dr. Alexander at Physicians' Hospital for another nerve block. That failed too. He has attempted to work with Dr. Doenitz to give me pain medication, but unfortunately causalgia doesn't respond to pain medication. So what they try to do is to numb my nerves as much as possible through medication. They really can't stop the pain, though."

The four defense attorneys objected.

Mike continued to question his client, ignoring them. "Mrs. Huffman, after February 1970 were you hospitalized? And, if so, why?"

"I was hospitalized at the Cliffs Hospital on June 17, 1970. Dr. Buchanan cut out two lymph nodes. A few days after that he removed my ovaries. The ovaries cause the body to manufacture the hormone estrogen, and the estrogen was feeding the malignancy in the lymph nodes—my malignancy is one that is estrogen-dependent."

"I object to that and ask that it be stricken," Arnold persisted.

Baylor also felt compelled to say, "I join in that. Obviously hearsay."

Mike continued to direct questions to his client. "Would you describe for us, Mrs. Huffman, the pain in your shoulder as it existed from April, 1970, to the present?"

Kathryn looked around the room to see if any of the defendants' attorneys were about to interrupt her, then answered slowly, "The pain ranges anywhere from a dull ache to a sharp shooting feeling. It could be like a knife cutting or somebody grabbing my shoulder. The pain travels all through my arm. The best way I can describe it is to tell you I've wanted to die because of it. It was . . . it *is* intolerable! I've attempted suicide because of the pain."

"I move that that answer be stricken. It goes into something that doesn't describe the pain," Baylor shouted.

"I join in that," Arnold said.

"I object also," Griffiths said.

Everyone turned to Ressler, who looked at each of his fellow attorneys and then said, "I join in that."

Mike went on, seemingly unperturbed by their objections. "Would you tell us the circumstances, Mrs. Huffman, that led up to the first time you tried to take your own life?"

"I object to the form of the question," Arnold said, leading off the objections.

The defendants' lawyers were becoming greatly agitated in their attempts to keep the plaintiff's comments off the record. "I so move. I'm sorry, but. . . ." Baylor was having difficulty completing his sentence.

"Continue, please," Mike said reassuringly to Kathryn.

Kathryn went calmly on. "On November 11, 1970, the lymph nodes under my arm were removed at Memorial Hospital. They were examined and found to be malignant. I had to take radioactive cobalt treatments—thirty-two altogether. There were two series: one in July, the other in December."

"Would you describe the cobalt treatment for us?"

"Well, first it meant going to New York to Dr. Norman Hastings' office every day, five days a week, for sixteen treatments. For the treatment itself, you lie down on a slab, and cobalt radiation is directed at your body."

"Is there any pain involved in that, either during or after the treatment?"

"Yes, there is. In the beginning there is a great deal of nausea and burning. Your skin gets scaly, and you have adhesions. Dr. Hastings and Dr. Doenitz told me that adhesions and scarring occur over the nerve endings. That makes the cobalt treatment very painful—very!"

"I ask that be stricken. An improper reply," Baylor said, putting his glasses down and fiddling with his pipe.

Mike acted as if he had not heard him. "Mrs. Huffman, would you tell us what you felt, if anything, as a result of the cobalt treatments?"

"Pain! A great deal of agonizing pain—aching, grabbing, shooting pains throughout my arm and shoulder."

"Was there any difference in how you felt after the July series of cobalt treatments and the way you felt after the December series?"

"The last treatments in December were worse."

"Would you tell us how? Was it different in degree or different in type of pain?"

"I was far more nauseated and enervated by the December treatments than by the July treatments."

"Would you tell us what you mean by enervated?"

"Very weak, finding it difficult to function, difficult to get around, to do anything; tired, worn out."

"How is your condition now as compared with this time last year, that is, in January of 1970?"

"There are times I have pain which is just as excruciating as it was last year. I just try to hang on."

She paused before continuing. "That's about all I can do—just hang on. The pain now keeps me from doing any work at the University. I had to refuse a professorship at the college where I'd been teaching because I can't stay on my feet for any period of time. I can hardly do anything because of the pain I have."

Mike said, "In addition to the treatments from the physicians you have testified about, are you receiving any other type of assistance or help at this time? And, if so, what? I'm not now referring or limiting the question to medical treatment."

"I just began to undergo rehabilitation therapy at the Rehabilitation Institute in New York."

"Is there an address that you can give us?" Arnold asked tartly, "and the name of the doctor you saw there?"

"Of course," Kathryn answered. "The doctor I saw there was Dr. Martin Feuss. The address is 88 Fifth Avenue, in New York."

"You have already had two appointments at the Rehabilitation Institute?" Mike asked.

"Yes."

"What was done during those two appointments?"

"They have a physical therapist who has been moving my arm and hand around and showing me a few exercises to do at home. They try to get my arm and hand moving."

"Would you tell us how the left arm compares with the right arm in size at the present time?" asked Mike.

"It's at least twice as large near my hand. I keep it wrapped with an elastic bandage. If it weren't wrapped, it would be much more swollen. It's extremely heavy and a dead weight. I wanted it to be amputated. . . ."

"Are you able to drop your left arm down to your side?"

"No. My elbow won't straighten out."

"Mrs. Huffman, I show you a photograph."

"What is the date of that photograph?" Baylor demanded.

Mike finished his sentence as if he hadn't heard. ". . . which was initialed by me on the back and dated July 23, 1970. Do you recall that as the first day you came to my office in Newark?" Mike passed the picture to Kathryn.

Kathryn took the picture and studied it. "Yes."

"And this photograph dated October 20, 1970, in which you are demonstrating your left arm; do you recall that photograph being taken in my office?" he asked as he showed Kathryn the other picture.

"Yes, I do."

"And these other photographs. Do you recall when they were taken at my office?" Mike asked, handing her several more.

"Yes," she replied after she had looked at each one of them.

"When were these taken?" Mike asked her.

"Today."

"Would you indicate for the record who took them and with what camera?" Griffiths said to Mike.

"These photographs were taken by me with a Polaroid camera," Mike stated.

"Mrs. Huffman, in the last photograph, does that show the farthest extent to which you can straighten out your left arm?"

"Yes, it does."

"And this photograph is another view?"

"Yes, sir."

"I have no further questions," Mike said as he nodded approvingly at his client.

Arnold got to his feet. "I have one question," he said.

"I'm going to have more than one, but go ahead," said Baylor, slouching down in his chair.

Arnold approached Kathryn. "Mrs. Huffman, when you had occasion to see Dr. Canaris on August 5, 1968, did the doctor examine both of your breasts?"

"Yes, he did."

"At that time was there anything called to your attention because of that examination as being abnormal?"

"No. He said I was perfectly healthy."

Arnold sat down.

Baylor took his time getting up from his chair, picked up some papers from the table, then walked slowly toward Kathryn.

"When you first talked to Dr. Lawrence and he gave you the prescription for The Pill, did he tell you what you could expect in the way of physical effects at that time?"

"He did."

"What did he tell you, please?"

"He told me headaches, nausea. . . ."

"Anything else?"

"Acne and sore breasts."

"Mrs. Huffman, please, just listen carefully to my question. Isn't it true that the only side effects that you can remember him telling you that you were going to get were headaches and an upset stomach? Isn't that so?"

Mike was annoyed by Baylor's line of questioning. "You are arguing with the witness, Mr. Baylor. The witness has answered your question with what she remembers. I object to the repetition of the question."

Baylor did not look at Mike as he was speaking, but waited impatiently for him to finish before going on.

"Were you aware of the risks of the side effects from oral contraceptives before you began taking them?"

Challenging Mr. Baylor's steel gaze with her own, Kathryn responded slowly and deliberately, "Dr. Lawrence only warned me about the minor side effects I just mentioned."

"Thank you, that's all I have," Baylor said, going back to his chair.

Ressler jumped up as Baylor finished. "I have a couple of questions," he said. He waved a small container in the air. "Did you, Mrs. Huffman, send a box of Mordrine pills to Dr. Canaris: a dispenser with pills that you got at Van's Pharmacy?"

"I did not send any pills to Dr. Canaris," Kathryn replied.

Ressler held up some notes, along with the pill box. "You did send this box to Dr. Canaris, did you not? Were there only twenty pills in it?" he asked as though Kathryn had not replied to his first question.

"I know positively that I did not send any *pills* to Dr. Canaris. I did fill the roulette-like Mordrine pill dispenser with candy mints and sent it off to Dr. Canaris. I wanted to make a very important point." Kathryn paused deliberately—"that birth control pills were being dispensed like candy."

"Thank you," Ressler said and returned to his seat.

Griffiths pushed his chair aside. "Now, it's my turn again, Mrs. Huffman," he said. "How did you go about getting a prescription for the birth control pills after you had the radical mastectomy?" he asked. "I mean the pills you emptied out of the container you sent Dr. Canaris."

"I just called up my internist and asked him for a prescription. He told me to pick it up at the drugstore."

"Did you tell him why you wanted them, what you planned to use the birth control pill container for?"

"No, the subject never came up."

"Did you call and tell him you wanted birth control pills for yourself?"

"I called him and said, 'Dr. Read, I would like some birth

control pills.' He said, 'Tell your pharmacist to phone me and I'll prescribe some Mordrine for you.' That was it.''

"Okay," Griffiths said. "Thank you." He sat down.

Mike looked around at the group of lawyers. "Any more questions?" he asked.

The lawyers shook their heads.

"Thank you for coming to my office, gentlemen. Good day." Mike stood up, dismissing them.

Kathryn sat still, watching each lawyer prepare to leave, while their assistants picked up the notes scattered over the big table.

The court reporter slowly put his equipment away. After the last lawyer left, he turned to Kathryn, "Good-bye and God bless you," he said.

Part Three

"... Although promoters of The Pill had the earliest and largest clinical experiences with The Pill . . . they were not the ones who discovered and reported serious adverse findings.

"Apparently, what was not looked for was not found. What was not surveyed was not seen. What perhaps happened was ignored. . . .

"To ignore the patients who dropped out was the radical failure of the highly touted and highly publicized study. . . . The researchers only studied women who had been on The Pill 25 months, which meant that any woman who had died before 25 months was not part of the study, nor were the "51 percent" of the women who dropped out the first 12 months because of complications. . . .

. . . This study lulled the medical profession into a false sense of security in respect to the safety of The Pill.

"I would like to conclude this section by saying that the social engineers *i.e.*, the population experts, in promoting The Pill regardless of safety are practicing chemical warfare on the women of this country."

Herbert Ratner, M.D.
Editor, Child & Family Quarterly
The Medical Hazards of the Birth Control Pill
Child and Family Reprint Booklet
Oak Park, Illinois 1969

Chapter One

Later that evening, January 16, 1971.
    Admission Date: 1/16/71

                        HUFFMAN, Kathryn Stuart
    Mrs. Huffman was admitted to The Cliffs Hospital as
an emergency patient. It was determined to initiate an
intensive course of chemotherapy.
    The patient did not respond well to the treatment. She
was on the critical list for 35 days and in isolation for the
duration of her hospitalization. Blood cell reduction was
reduced to the fullest extent in an attempt to effect a state
of remission. 2/20/71, the patient fell and sustained a
fractured nose while trying to get into a wheelchair to
return home.

                        Herman Doenitz, M.D.
    Discharge Date: 2/20/71

January 26, 1971.
    Mike sent Kathryn a copy of a letter he wrote to Paul Slater.

    Depositions are now scheduled as follows: Drs.
Lawrence and Canaris will be deposed at 2 P.M., January
27th, at Baylor's office in Jersey City.

I'm sending a copy of this letter to Kathryn. I'll leave it up to her whether or not she wants to attend their depositions. She has the right to attend, but there is no obligation.

Kathryn was unable to attend the doctors' depositions. She was on the critical list.

February 26, 1971.
Kathryn received a letter from Mike Jefferson.

Dear Kathryn:
Paul Slater and I have discussed the importance that you execute a Will in order to prevent your interest in the litigation from reverting to your husband. We have received several substantial offers from the drug companies as well as the physicians' lawyers to settle this case out of court.
I urge you to take steps in this connection at the earliest possible time with your local attorney. I would be glad to assist, if necessary.

March 2, 1971.
Sam Groden came to her bedside at home. Kathryn told him what to put in her Will:
"I give my entire residuary estate which I may own or to which I may be entitled at the time of my death to my parents, Noreen and Roy Stuart. If they do not survive me, I bequeath my estate to my beloved grandmother, Kathryn Windsor.
"I specifically have failed to make provision in this, my last Will and Testament, for my husband, Conrad Huffman."

March 22, 1971.
This was the day Kathryn was to appear in court in New York City for her divorce. Her doctors tried to prevail upon her not to go.

Doctors Engle and Doenitz had wanted to give her medication that would lower her level of consciousness, as she had entered the most distressing phase of her illness.

"I'll not permit it," Kathryn insisted. "I must remain alert and rational at least until I finish what I've set out to do."

She painstakingly dressed herself. She put on a light-yellow pleated wool skirt and a short yellow cut-away jacket. Her blouse was white cotton printed with yellow roses. The yellow rose, the official flower of Texas, where she was born, was Kathryn's favorite flower. Her wedding bouquet had been yellow roses, and the orchestra had serenaded her by playing "The Yellow Rose of Texas" during the wedding dinner.

"Ready?" her father asked as he entered her room.

"I was just thinking about my wedding—and you ask if I'm ready to leave for my divorce! How's that for a coincidence?"

Without waiting for her father's reply, she eased her left arm into a yellow silk scarf made into a sling. With a look of complete confidence she left home for the first time in a month.

Len and Irv Ingram, her divorce attorneys, were awaiting Kathryn at the courthouse. They gave her a few instructions and suggested that she sit on the left side of the courtroom. Her parents were seated behind her.

Soon Judge Branas entered the courtroom. Kathryn's attorneys took their seats before the judge, where Conrad's lawyer was also seated.

Kathryn was called to the stand first.

While she was being sworn in, Judge Branas was observing her. He looked at Conrad, who was seated next to his parents, then at Kathryn's parents. He thumbed through some papers.

Quite suddenly, Judge Branas stopped the proceedings and told the lawyers to meet with him in his chambers. Kathryn was asked to step down.

A short time later, the clerk of the court came over to her.

"Judge Branas would like you and your parents to go to Room 735," he said.

Room 735 was near the courtroom and had the judge's name on the door. Kathryn, her mother, and her father had waited there a few minutes when a nurse appeared.

"I've been asked to see that you be made as comfortable as possible," she said to Kathryn. "Why don't you lie down on this couch, if you wish, and I'll get you a pillow."

Kathryn didn't hesitate; she immediately collapsed on the couch.

"Please," she whispered, "give me an injection." In addition to her usual pain, she seemed to have great difficulty breathing.

An hour later, her attorneys appeared. Len leaned over her as she rested on the couch, and whispered, "It's all over, Kathryn."

Kathryn opened her eyes and looked at him in wonder.

"Over?" she asked.

"Yes, it's unbelievable! The judge was absolutely enraged about the divorce action. He said that he wished this could be tried as a criminal case, because he would like to lock Conrad up for good!"

April 13, 1971. Home of the Stuarts.

Kathryn's breathing became more difficult. Her parents took her to Dr. Doenitz's office. The doctor explained that the area around Kathryn's heart had filled with fluid and could result in heart failure if it wasn't drained. The procedure he explained was simple. A tube was to be inserted into her left lung which would drain out the fluid. She was coughing, and that, Dr. Doenitz said, was because of a change in the tissue of her left lung as a result of the cobalt therapy. It was the cobalt therapy that had caused the fluid to gather in the sac around her heart. He said he would make the necessary arrangements for the drainage procedure and advised that she be admitted to the Cliffs Hospital immediately.

Later that day.

Kathryn was surprised to get a telephone call from a well-known figure in Washington, D.C., who was "quietly" collecting material regarding The Pill. He had learned of her case and asked her to send him an affidavit regarding the circumstances under which The Pill had been prescribed for her. She sent a copy of the letter to Mike:

> My name is Kathryn Stuart Huffman, and I live at 9306 Crawford Road in Short Hills, New Jersey. I am submitting this affidavit to state that I would not have used oral contraceptives if it had not been for the assurance of two physicians that this birth control procedure was the safest and best for my health. I further swear to the fact that had the true nature of the medication been made known to me, I would have never taken the birth control pill.

The affidavit continued with the full history of her case.

Evening, April 13, 1971.
    Admitted 4:00 P.M.

                              Kathryn Stuart Huffman
                              Cliffs Hospital #72194
    The attempt to drain the patient's lung without giving her an anesthetic failed. The pain was so severe when the resident attempted to insert the tube that she would not let him continue. . . .

That evening, Kathryn and Dr. Engle discussed this matter and arrangements were made to have Dr. Kellerman anesthetize her while a surgeon friend of Dr. Engle inserted the tube into her lung. The surgery was scheduled for April 16.

April 16, 1971. Cliffs Hospital.
    Kathryn was burning with fever.
    "I simply must have some water," she said.
    "Sorry, dear. No water before the anesthesia," the nurse told her.

Kathryn closed her eyes. She mumbled as if she were not entirely conscious.

"Kathryn," a voice said. It was Dr. Engle. "Kathryn, I just learned that your divorce was finalized. You're legally back to being Kathryn Stuart!"

He then went into the adjoining bathroom and returned with a cold, wet towel. He placed the cool cloth on Kathryn's burning cheeks, then let her suck the cloth.

Several nurses arrived with a rolling table and wheeled Kathryn out of her room. Dr. Engle took her hand as he accompanied her into the operating room.

She was returned to her hospital room two hours later. There was a tube in her back with liquid draining from it into a jar.

Kathryn's parents sat quietly at her bedside. At about 9:55 P.M. Dr. Doenitz appeared. He asked Noreen and Roy to join him in the waiting room.

"Your daughter is in a coma," he said quietly. "She will not regain consciousness. . . . I'm sorry. . . . I'm sure you don't want her to suffer anymore. . . ."

Just at that moment, an announcement was made on the television, "It's 10:00 P.M. Do you know where your children are?"

Noreen bolted out of the waiting room and ran to Kathryn in utter panic. Dr. Engle was standing by Kathryn's bedside. He took Noreen's hand and gently led her into the hall. "Do have the courage to go on," he said. "Kathryn is counting on you to carry on for her. . . ."

Roy and Dr. Doenitz caught up to her. Roy put his arm around Noreen and they returned to Kathryn's bedside.

Noreen gazed out the window around 2:00 A.M. She suddenly noticed that the sky was filled with hundreds of stars. They were shining brightly as if they were rejoicing. She noticed that Kathryn's breathing was becoming faint. Kathryn's classical beauty had remained untouched by this terrible disease that had ravaged her body. Noreen detected a smile on her lips. . . .

Dr. Doenitz appeared and briefly examined Kathryn. As Noreen embraced her daughter with her eyes, the doctor put his arm around her.

"Kathryn is gone. . . ." he said.

From the Record

NEW JERSEY STATE DEPARTMENT OF HEALTH						

LOCAL FILE NUMBER — **CERTIFICATE OF DEATH** — STATE FILE NUMBER

SPACES BELOW FOR STATE USE ONLY	1. NAME OF DECEASED (Type or Print) (First) Kathryn (Middle) Stuart (Last) Huffman	2. Sex F	3. DATE OF DEATH 4-17-71

PLACE — 4. Color or Race **White** — 5. Age (in yrs. last birthday) **25** / Months / Days / Hours / Min. — 6. Date of Birth **11-7-1945** — 7. Was deceased ever in U.S. Armed Forces? (Yes, no, or unknown) (If yes, give war or dates of serv.) **NO** **NO**

8. Birthplace (State or foreign country) **Texas** — 9. Citizen of what country? **U S A** — 10. Married ☐ Never Married ☐ Widowed ☐ Divorced ☒ — 11. Social Security No. **Not available**

RESIDENCE — 12. PLACE OF DEATH — a. County **Bergen** — 13. USUAL RESIDENCE (If institution: residence before admission) a. State **N.J.** b. County **Essex**

b. City ☒ Boro ☐ Twp ☐ **Englewood** — c. City ☐ Boro ☐ Twp ☒ **Short Hills**

c. Name of (If not in hospital or institution give street address) Hospital or Institution **Cliffs Hospital** — d. Street Address (If rural, P.O. Address) **9306 Crawford Rd., Short Hills**

14. a. Usual Occupation (Give kind of work done during most of working life, even if retired) **Doctoral Student** — 14. b. Kind of Business or Industry **None**

15. Father's Name **Roy Stuart** — 16. Mother's Maiden Name **Noreen Windsor**

17. Informant's Name and Address **Roy Stuart, 9306 Crawford Rd., Short Hills, N.J.**

CAUSE — 18. PART I DEATH WAS CAUSED BY — Enter only one cause per line for (a), (b) and (c) — Approximate interval between onset and death

Immediate Cause (a) *Respiratory Failure* — *1 week*

Conditions, if any, which gave rise to above cause (a), stating the underlying cause last — Due to (b) *Lung and Pleural Metastases* — *3 months*

Due to (c) *Breast Cancer* — *21 months*

PART II OTHER SIGNIFICANT CONDITIONS — 19a. Was autopsy — 19b. If yes, were findings considered

"If I must die . . . and die so terribly . . . , at least let me die feeling fulfilled.

"I want to feel I've done everything I could to expose this secrecy of silence that exists about The Pill.

"I want to warn others—so they won't be misinformed or have to suffer the pain and agony I've had. . . ."

Epilogue

May 10, 1972.

The trial against the two pharmaceutical companies and the two doctors was scheduled to begin on this date. Kathryn's mother was the "substitute" plaintiff for her deceased daughter.

One of Kathryn's closest friends, Sarah Neumann, was to stand in for Kathryn on the witness stand. Sarah had a bound copy of Kathryn's testimony, taken during the deposition, and she held it tightly. Sarah's parents were both physicians. The negligence demonstrated by Kathryn's doctors distressed them deeply. Sarah, like Kathryn, was receiving her doctorate in international law. She shared Kathryn's ideals; she was determined to carry on for her friend. She had pressed a yellow rose in the last page of the thick deposition. She sat between Kathryn's parents in the rear of the courtroom, staring at the defendants, whom she blamed for her friend's horrible, untimely death.

Kathryn's lawyers, Mike Jefferson and Paul Slater, were seated in front of the room near the witness stand. They had dozens of books and documents on the table before them. Four junior lawyers from their law firms were seated directly behind them. Slater, who practiced in New York, had qualified to practice in New Jersey especially for Kathryn's case.

Seated to the left of Mike and Paul were the defendants'

lawyers. Baylor and Griffiths represented the manufacturers. Arnold and Ressler were seated next to their physician clients, Dr. Lawrence and Dr. Canaris, who were being sued for negligence. About a dozen junior lawyers accompanied the four senior attorneys.

Thirty possible jurors were gathered in the middle of the courtroom. They whispered among themselves as they looked around the room.

At the back of the room, a middle-aged woman sat by herself. She had a briefcase on the floor by her side, and a yellow pad in her lap.

Some twenty physicians were prepared to testify as "expert" witnesses. Dr. Frank Gawron, a leading specialist in the treatment of breast cancer, was to testify that women who got breast cancer after taking The Pill had a more aggressive and rapidly developing cancer than those women who did not take The Pill. It was his opinion that The Pill shortened Kathryn's life by many years and it was possible that the "seed" of cancer might never have been stimulated to grow without The Pill. He felt the speed with which the cancer grew and spread had been the result of The Pill. Because the cancer was so vicious and aggressive it intensified Kathryn's pain and suffering.

Dr. Julius Wilkinson, the surgeon who performed Kathryn's radical mastectomy, wanted to testify on her behalf. Still badly shaken by what happened to Kathryn, he felt he should pursue her cause. He was prepared to testify that after her breast was removed, the pathologists' reports did not show any spread of cancer. The analysis of the breast tissues indicated she had the type of breast cancer that was least likely to have spread. Yet, some two and a half years later she died from the spread of the cancer. In his deposition, Wilkinson had explained at some length how estrogen, contained in The Pill, can alter the appearance of breast cancer. This concerned him—he said Kathryn had the "strangest" tumor he ever saw. He was also prepared to discuss the course of the problems Kathryn had because the wound took so long to heal.

A second surgeon, Dr. Robert Buchanan, was to testify on Kathryn's behalf. He was the surgeon who first detected the cancer spread and determined that she had an estrogen-dependent malignancy. He then removed her ovaries to try to reduce the amount of estrogen in her body—to no avail. Since The Pill contained estrogen, he felt that it most certainly cut her life span short and altered the course of the disease.

Dr. Herman Doenitz, Kathryn's cancer internist, was to testify that nothing could slow down the course of the disease. Thirty-two cobalt treatments and powerful chemotherapy failed to help. He was unable to relieve her pain even though he gave her the strongest possible medication.

Dr. Alvin Engle, the neurologist, would also take the stand. He wanted it to be a matter of record that Kathryn was an exceptional young woman in every way, anticipating that the defendants' lawyers might try to present her in an unfavorable light. In his own deposition he said, "Despite this very gloomy situation, Kathryn displayed a stable and determined personality profile." He also was prepared to discuss fully that she was in a state of "constant and continual agony" due to pain and swelling.

If there was any challenge that Kathryn lacked the intellectual ability to understand the pros and cons of taking The Pill if her doctors had presented them, that assumption could easily be destroyed. One of Kathryn's professors, a leading international political scientist, was eager to expose the undemocratic processes that existed within institutions and "privileged" groups. In his deposition, he said that Kathryn was "a brilliant student who was slated to have an outstanding career in her chosen field." He was prepared to discuss the excellent relationships she had with her friends and teachers at the University. Also, Kathryn's deposition and affidavit were to be used as evidence that she would *not* have taken The Pill had she been given the "bad news" about it.

Dr. Anthony Gable was to testify that the drug companies failed to furnish the physicians with adequate warnings in the package insert and other literature.

At 9:30 A.M., Judge Donald Wilcox came out of his chambers. The bailiff rapped his gavel and told everyone to rise.

Soon after the session began, Baylor addressed the court and requested that the selection of jurors be postponed. He wanted first to establish what parts of the testimony from Kathryn's deposition would be admissible. For that, all potential jurors were asked to leave the room. The judge listened as Baylor argued that some of Kathryn's comments, which Sarah would repeat on the witness stand, should be omitted.

The judge, an impressive, handsome, middle-aged man, asked the attorney to read the portions he wanted stricken. Baylor said, "I asked her to tell us how she felt emotionally. She replied, 'Emotionally? I'll tell you, Mr. Baylor. You probably saved my life last night, or prolonged it, whatever. I would have killed myself if it weren't that I was going to appear here for the deposition today. . . .'" Baylor continued to read the passage to its conclusion, where Kathryn accused him of harassing her, "'I might not be alive when the judge reviews this record, Mr. Baylor, but I know he will agree with me and let the record stand. . . .'"

The judge looked at Baylor and said, "Her answers were responsive to your questions. They will remain as her testimony."

Baylor's aplomb vanished. He looked at the judge in disbelief.

"Your honor," Arnold said, "I'd like to have the decedent's comments stricken regarding Dr. Lawrence. In her deposition she said, 'I didn't want to use Dr. Lawrence anymore. He'd been rather crude in his speech.'" He continued with Kathryn's comments on what Lawrence had said and that he had "misrepresented The Pill."

The judge addressed Arnold. "Her comments will remain. From what she said, this Dr. Lawrence did appear to be a rather crude doctor and not such a good one. Her reply was responsive."

Arnold paled as Ressler jumped up. "Your honor," he said, a tremor of rage in his voice, "I move to have the decedent's comments stricken regarding my client, Dr. Vittorio Canaris. She testified in the deposition 'He [Dr. Canaris] suggested that perhaps the reason I was complaining about so many side effects was that I was dubious about taking The Pill and these side effects were in fact products of my imagination, rather than really caused by The Pill. . . . And then he assumed I was frigid with my husband because I was "up tight" during the internal examination.' "

The judge glared at Ressler. "Your motion to strike her response is denied." At this, the middle-aged woman who had been sitting alone at the back of the room closed her briefcase with a snap, rose, and walked out of the courtroom. Immediately, Griffiths, one of the drug companies' lawyers, jumped up and asked for a thirty-minute recess. The judge agreed.

As the judge walked back to his chambers, Baylor and Griffiths left the courtroom in great haste. As they opened the door, the woman could be seen, obviously waiting for them. Arnold and Ressler remained behind, slouched on the hard bench. Soon, Baylor appeared at the door and called the remaining senior attorneys to join them outside the courtroom. Some twenty minutes later, the defendants' lawyers appeared and beckoned to Mike Jefferson and Paul Slater.

In five minutes, Mike and Paul re-entered the courtroom and approached Kathryn's parents and Sarah.

"That woman who just went out," Paul said, "is from Lloyds of London. She's here because her company covers a part of the damages the drug companies would have to pay. She's been talking with the attorneys, and they say they want to settle before the jury is selected."

Noreen gasped. "Settle! But we've carried this fight— Kathryn's fight—"

"We know how you feel, Noreen," Paul interrupted gently. "You want to carry it through to the end, for Kathryn's sake. We understand that. But today Kathryn had her day in court.

"Having the jury find the two doctors and the drug firms guilty isn't the primary reason Kathy initiated this lawsuit. It was to change the way that drugs are disseminated and to show the harm that medical technology can do. As far as we know, hers will be the first Pill-related breast cancer case to be settled *in* court. The effect will be exactly the same as if we went to trial.

"That woman from Lloyd's is a sign of things to come. The insurance companies aren't going to let this kind of arrogance and hanky-panky by drug firms and doctors continue. They can't afford to! And that, after all, is what we wanted to accomplish. That's why Mike and I strongly recommend that you settle."

Noreen looked at Mike pleadingly. "I promised Kathryn before she died that I'd make her experiences public, just the way they're described in the deposition. I will *not* go back on my promise to her!"

"The terms of the agreement would be that the amount of the settlement and the names of the parties involved in the suit not be disclosed. So long as the real names aren't mentioned, or the amount of the settlement, there's no reason you can't make Kathryn's story public," Mike reassured her.

Paul nodded in agreement. "The trial could go on for several months. Every day would be a fresh pain for you and Roy—for all of you who loved Kathryn. You've been through so much already."

Noreen hesitated. She had to rely on her lawyer's advice.

"Noreen," Mike added, "you know Kathryn wouldn't have wanted the people she loved to go through that agony, not when you can accomplish the same thing without it."

It was true. Reluctantly, Noreen agreed to settle. The avalanche had begun to move; it was a handful of pebbles now, but leaders in every area of specialization had vowed to carry on for Kathryn. With their help, the mountain of secrecy would crumble.

Kathryn's successful case against incompetence and secrecy in the field of medicine opened the door to many more efforts. Through them, the public is growing alert to the dangers of indiscriminate pill-taking, and the pill-dealing of our modern medicine men.

The "conspiracy of silence" among drug companies, the medical profession, and government agencies that has existed over the years still exists but it is being exposed. According to a report by medical writer Justin Faherty of *The Record*, ". . . a damaging aspect came to light last month with the revelation that thousands of suits against the seven U.S. manufacturers of oral contraceptives have been kept under wraps through secrecy agreements as a precondition to cash settlements." In his article dated January 29, 1975, he referred to a story revealing that "constitutional experts and public-interest lawyers claim that a second device to assure secrecy—'sealing the file'—keeps the public from learning of problems associated with The Pill."

In November, 1975, *Newsweek* published an article called "Perils of the Pill," in which it reported that a number of researchers had suspected for a long time that there was a connection between the contraceptive pill and breast cancer, but their suspicions had been based on animal research. Now, however, a report on the largest study so far, the result of an investigation in California, based on use by women, suggests a connection, at least for some women. The article concludes that women who use The Pill before having children and women with a history of benign breast tumors who use The Pill "face a heightened risk of malignancy."

In a cancer-conscious society, can one justify "heightening the risk" of breast cancer? Breast cancer occurs in one out of ten women whose mother, maternal aunt or sister had breast cancer. This disease does not need to be promoted—it needs to be extinguished.

Dr. Herbert Ratner reported to the Senate Subcommittee that, as of 1970, 8,500,000 women were reported to have 6,561,500 disease conditions due to The Pill. Why has this dangerous drug been so imprudently promoted?

The population explosion: The emphasis has been placed on population control rather than on the health of the individual. The birth rate should not be controlled by killing potential mothers or creating a sick society.

Incompetent medical care: February 1, 1976, *The New York*

Times reported in an article entitled, "U.S. Doctors: About 5 Percent Are Unfit":

> . . . Part of the drug reactions problem can be traced to the bewildering variety of drugs available to doctors. About 1200 different drugs are on the market, many more than any doctor can possibly know well. No drug is completely safe, all have potential side effects, each is intended for a specific use. Yet any licensed doctor is free to use any drug in any way he cares to, regardless of how well or how long ago he has been trained or how diligently or poorly he keeps his knowledge up to date. . . .
>
> . . . Advocates of regulatory reform say medicine's disciplinary bodies have remained weak because of the professional veil of silence that commonly shields serious incidents from outside attention and because of the difficulty of getting patients to complain and testify against their doctors. Lately more attention has been focused on the deficiencies of medical practice as the result of two forces. One is the growing involvement of the Federal government in paying for health services. The other is the rise of the consumer movement, which has stimulated activists, including conscientious doctors, to seek and disclose hitherto obscure information.

Money: According to Morton Mintz in his book, *The Pill: An Alarming Report*, one pharmaceutical company made $147,700,000 from sales of The Pill and of estrogen to "stay young." This was in 1968 when "only" an estimated seven million women took The Pill, compared to an estimated ten million today.

The pharmaceutical companies seem to have a financial investment in doctors. Mintz reported in his book, ". . . though it is widely known that the drug industry is consistently the nation's most profitable, it is not generally grasped that the profitability is tied to an expenditure for promotion and advertising of $4500 per physician per year, according to an estimate in 1968 of the Prescription Drug Task Force of the Department of Health, Education and Welfare. This kind of money talks—and talks much more loudly than an occasional cautionary article in a medical or scientific journal. . . ."

February 10, 1976, *The New York Times* reported that pharmaceutical companies canceled a half-million dollars' worth of advertising in a magazine owned by The New York Times Company. This was in retaliation for *The New York Times* running the series on medical incompetence mentioned above. Reportedly, the advertisers warned an officer of the magazine, "You don't feed people who beat you up."

Boyce Rensberger of *The New York Times* reported that the American Association for the Advancement of Science was concerned about the quality of research being published. On February 2, 1975, he wrote, "Although outright frauds, such as the recent incident in which a cancer researcher faked his results, are considered rare, many scientists are becoming concerned with the tendency of some of their colleagues to exaggerate the conclusions that can be drawn from their experiments, especially if the exaggeration can bring popular acclaim or grant money. . . ."

Politics: The American Medical Association and the pharmaceutical companies have strong lobby groups. The political association between these two groups goes back as far as 1938, when the American Medical Association opposed legislation calling for the safety of drugs to be established before being sold to the public. David Burnham, a reporter for *The New York Times*, reported on July 20, 1975, that these two groups exchanged professional lobbyists. They recently have been linked together in "secret, successful drives to kill a bill aimed at reducing the costs of drugs."

Their political alliance appears to be intertwined with their financial interests. This is understandable for "big business." But can a physician follow the principle of his profession, *primum noli nocere*—first do no harm—and at the same time be indebted to a group whose stand is, "You don't feed people who beat you up"? If physicians' loyalties are going to conflict—between their patients and the big drug interests—then their patients had better be made aware of the doctors' new image.

Men: Millions of men have shirked their responsibility regarding birth control measures other than to demand that women use contraceptives. The question has been frequently raised whether this uncontrolled experiment with The Pill would have been conducted on ten million men.

Nicholas Von Hoffman, a reporter for *The Washington Post*, wrote, ". . . men's medical treatment of women isn't reassuring. On balance it appears hundreds of thousands of women have been given this drug without being told what's not yet known about it and often with assurances of safety which the evidence does not justify. . . .

". . . Men, especially in executive positions, will not even admit it is an issue, which isn't surprising in a sex that continues to believe it has a right to direct the most intimate functions of the other sex's body.

"Would we have the problem of The Pill or all this fuss and claptrap over abortions if it were men who got pregnant?"

Pregnancy: Dr. Ratner testified at the 1970 Senate hearing on The Pill, "The real panic makers are those supporters of The Pill who are trying to make The Pill appear safe by exaggerating the dangers of pregnancy. . . . Such dramatization, I assure you, is of no comfort to millions of women in the United States presently pregnant or considering pregnancy."

If a woman is postponing having a family, she should have second thoughts about the possible effects The Pill might have on her offspring even if she is not concerned about her own body.

Dr. Roy Hertz, in a contribution to the 1966 *FDA Report on the Oral Contraceptives*, reported, "An unequivocal abnormality produced by estrogen-progesterone combinations is the suppression of ovulation itself. It is only reasonable to consider the ultimate fate of the ovum that would have been normally released from the ovary. We do not know whether this ovum dies or survives. If it survives, is it altered in any way? . . . For an adequate analysis of this problem 100,000 children would be required . . . [and] these children would have to be followed for 6 to 9 years in order to completely appraise any possible effects upon them. . . .

"In view of the serious limitations in our knowledge of the potential long-term effects of estrogen-progesterone combinations, it is mandatory that further clinical experience be gained under properly controlled conditions of observation and follow-up."

In an effort to avoid pregnancies, The Pill has been given to tens of thousands of teenagers, some as young as 14 years old. Howie Kurtz, staff writer for *The Record*, reported that about 4,000 "kids" are seen each year at one of the four teen clinics in the Washington, D.C., area alone. The Pill is handed out like candy— and usually without parental consent—despite the fact that it is particularly dangerous at that age. Dr. Carl Djerassi, who synthesized the first pill, said in an interview for *Prism*, that it was not a good idea to "monkey around" with hormones during the teenage period.

Experimentation with humans: This massive uncontrolled experiment on 10 million woman was aptly summarized by Dr. Herbert Ratner, editor of the *Child and Family Quarterly* (1969):

"In an age in which preventive medicine has high priority, it is distressing to have women exploited as guinea pigs in order to establish absolute certitude of the causal relationship of The Pill to cancer and other complications. Though it must be admitted women make superb guinea pigs—they don't cost anything, feed themselves, clean their own 'cages', pay for their own pills and remunerate the clinical observer—the letter and spirit of the Kefauver Bill was to the contrary: that safety be established before, not after, placing the drugs on the market. . . .

". . . Human guinea pigs at no charge is an attractive gift to physicians doing clinical research. One would be happier, however, if these physicians displayed more of a public health conscience and raised their voices against a mass experiment proceeding more from ignorance than from knowledge."

Kathryn's story is told here in a personal way. Kathryn Huffman was a real person, with real feelings. She was not, however, treated as a "real" person. She was denied information she sought, and that denial in a democratic society made a mockery of the right of self-determination, the right to informed consent, the right to individual freedom of choice, and the right to knowledge. That denial was immoral and unethical on the part of all those who played a role in it.

Because Kathryn believed in the right to pursue knowledge, every dollar received from the settlement in her case was donated to various libraries. It was Kathryn's wish to make knowledge—knowledge of all kinds—more available to all.